Many people organising a research project need to know how many people they will likely have to recruit, but might not have ready access to a statistician. This book has been written to help them. It also contains an introduction to statistical ideas for people who have not studied the subject. It uses the method of programmed learning, making it suitable for people without a teacher to learn by themselves.

Miland Joshi took his MSc in Medical Statistics from Leicester and a PhD in Statistics in Warwick. A Chartered Statistician, he has taught and given statistical support to health professionals and other academics over two decades. He has served as a statistical advisor on a number of review committees for research applications. Some of the methods in this book were presented by the author as a guest speaker during the Upper Egypt Assisted Reproduction Symposium in 2024 for specialist physicians and surgeons.

How big should my sample be?
A Guide for Health Researchers

Miland Joshi

© Miland Joshi, 2024
All rights reserved.

Foreword

I am very pleased to write an endorsement for this book.

It is special because it has a very clear focus: to be a user-friendly text for non-statisticians who use statistics or are willing to start using statistics without a deep understanding of the topic.

The book is a simple guide through the most common statistical analysis techniques used in planning medical research projects, particularly clinical trials. It also has more advanced sections focused on the statistical methods commonly used in this area, making it a well-rounded and concise statistical text.

It introduces some basic but essential concepts, such as the normal distribution, to dive deep into more complex areas, such as study types, continuous and proportion outcomes, estimate precision, power calculations, equal and unequal arms and more.

Readers will find this book like a companion that will take them on a statistical journey without technical jargon but with very simple and real examples. It will enhance their comprehension of the simple and more complex concepts, specifically focusing on clinical trial statistics.

This book has many prompts to ensure the reader absorbs, reflects on, and applies statistical concepts and techniques using real-world examples to which the reader can relate.

Additionally, the author provides simple but clear examples of statistical calculations, aiming to reinforce the new knowledge the reader has acquired.

The specific sections on clinical trials are due to the author's expertise in this area. These sections are rich in examples to further enhance readers' comprehension of the topics.

I recommend this book as your new companion for your statistical journey.

Professor Andrea Manfrin
Visiting Professor in the School of Pharmacy and Biomedical Sciences
University of Central Lancashire

Preface

This book is intended to be a guide to researchers who are not statisticians, particularly health professionals or scientists, in designing their projects, particularly clinical trials. It is intended primarily as a teaching book, using the well-known method of programmed instruction. Given its intended readers, it does not go into mathematical details found in textbooks for aspiring professional Statisticians such as Matthews (2006), although some details are given for reference in a technical Appendix. It should be possible to work through this book with only a simple calculator that can do basic arithmetic.

The book aims to provide basic training and knowledge only. It does not deal with more advanced topics, such as cross-over studies, or outcome measurements with unusual distributions, that may need computer simulation. It is not a substitute for encyclopaedic works like Julious (2023), or specialised articles in scientific journals, found in university libraries. It may, however, be a genuine help to researchers who wish to plan fairly simple studies, but who do not have ready access to a statistician.

Acknowledgments

I would like to thank a number of people. Professor Emeritus John Whitehead for his good teaching and encouragement for the idea of an effort at public statistical education.

Professor Andrea Manfrin for writing the foreword, and Mr Dudley Gentles, Professor Stephen Bremner and Dr. Shaheen Tonse for looking over the manuscript and making helpful suggestions and corrections. Mrs Fleur Dorrell for arranging contact with the artist, and help with the back cover text.

Ms Tiana Dunlop for an attractive cover design, which I could never have dreamed up. I'm happy to help artists by saying that book authors do well to seek their services for the presentation of their work.

Last, but not least - on the contrary, most of all - I, the author, would like to thank my parents for a lifetime of generosity on their part.

Contents

1 Introduction   **1**
  1.1 General Aims 1
  1.2 The method we use 1
  1.3 What we cover 2

2 Statistical Ideas   **5**
  2.1 Data 5
  2.2 Populations and Samples 6
  2.3 The Normal distribution 8
  2.4 Samples are not all the same 9
  2.5 Confidence Intervals 10
  2.6 Statistical tests 11
  2.7 Power 11
  2.8 Sample size 12
  2.9 Precision 13
  2.10 Correlation 13
  2.11 Prevalence and Incidence 14
  2.12 Randomized Clinical Trials 15
  2.13 Diagnostic test studies 17
  2.14 Epidemiological studies 18
  2.15 Preliminary studies 18
  2.16 Looking ahead 19

3 Preliminary studies   21
3.1 Context 21
3.2 Dose finding studies 22
3.3 Feasibility studies 23
3.4 Pilot studies 24

4 Two arms   27
4.1 Types of outcome 27
4.2 Caution about assuming Normality . 28
4.3 Continuous Outcomes 29
4.4 Proportions 31
    4.4.1 Proportions not in the table . 33
    4.4.2 Survival studies 34
4.5 Allowing for dropouts 35
4.6 Hedging your bets 37
4.7 Research Ethics committees 39

5 Precision   41

6 Optional topics   45
6.1 Multiple testing 45
6.2 Unequal arms 46
6.3 Compliance 48
    6.3.1 A note on analysis 48
    6.3.2 A note on policy 49
6.4 Clusters 49
6.5 Rule of 3 for rare events 51
    6.5.1 Application to Diagnostic Tests 52
6.6 Rule of 10 for Epidemiology 54
6.7 Before-after correlation 56
6.8 Incidence rates 57
6.9 Non-inferiority trials 60
    6.9.1 Continuous outcomes 60

	6.9.2 Proportions	61
6.10	Factorial trials	63

7 Revision Exercises — 65

7.1 Main topics — 65
    7.1.1 Two-arm trial: Continuous outcome — 65
    7.1.2 Two-arm trial: Proportions — 66
    7.1.3 Precision — 67

7.2 Optional topics — 67
    7.2.1 Multiple testing — 67
    7.2.2 Unequal arms — 68
    7.2.3 Compliance — 68
    7.2.4 Clusters — 69
    7.2.5 Rule of 3 for rare events: confidence interval — 70
    7.2.6 Rule of 3 for rare events: sample size — 70
    7.2.7 Diagnostic Tests — 71
    7.2.8 Rule of 10 for statistical modelling: sample size — 71
    7.2.9 Before-after correlation — 72
    7.2.10 Incidence rates — 72
    7.2.11 Non-inferiority trials: Continuous Outcomes — 73
    7.2.12 Non-inferiority trials: Proportions — 74
    7.2.13 Factorial trials — 74

Afterword — 76

Technical Appendix — 81

Bibliography

Chapter 1

Introduction

1.1 General Aims

This book aims to help you find a sample of sufficient size for answering your own scientific question. It is not intended to be the sort of encyclopaedic work or specialised text that you might find in university libraries. Nor is it a substitute for consulting a statistician. But it may help you find an answer to your question "How big should my sample be?"

1.2 The method we use

The method we use is called *programmed instruction*, which has been around for decades[1]. It presents you with a small amount of material, and then asks you a question. You need to answer the question before proceeding. We will indicate

---

[1] See, for example Rowntree (2018)

a question in *italics* with a line of stars following. Try to answer the question before proceeding. You might like to read with a piece of paper or card as you go along, to cover up the answer after the stars.

Q: Is this book intended to be a comprehensive textbook?

****

I hope you answered that this is not *intended to be a comprehensive textbook. It is intended to help people who could use guidance, but without having to go into technical details.*

1.3 What we cover

We begin with a chapter on elementary statistical ideas. This is not intended to be a complete account of the field at all, just a preparation for what follows. After that, successive chapters deal with the common situations for which you might need a sample size. The more important topics in this book include clinical trials where the outcome is measured on a scale, trials where the outcomes are proportions, and epidemiological studies where we want to measure a proportion with a required precision.

By the end of the book you should be in a good position to do sample size calculations for many of the common types of studies, though there will

1.3. WHAT WE COVER 3

certainly be more complex studies for which you will need to consult a statistician.

Chapter 2

Statistical Ideas

This chapter is intended to give you an understanding of some statistical ideas you need in order to understand the material that follows. It is not intended to be a complete account of Statistics. If you have already studied an elementary course in Statistics, you may well not need it, except as a quick refresher.

If you should feel the need for a proper book on Statistics but are put off the idea of large or technical works, I would recommend Rowntree (2018). It is very reader-friendly, and in fact Rowntree's method of programmed instruction is the method that we have tried to follow in this book.

2.1 Data

I'm sure you've seen the word *data* in many places. For our purposes it is *information in the form of numbers*. These may often be measurements on a scale, which may take any value, and so are called *continuous*, but they may also be *binary* measurements (0 or 1), in which we assign the value 1 to an individual if they fall in a certain group, and 0 otherwise. For example women might be given the code 1, and men 0.

Continuous measurements can be summarised using numbers called *statistics*. Two common ones are the *mean* or average, and the *standard deviation* or SD which is a measure of variability, that is, how spread out a set of observations is. Data can often be represented in pictures called *histograms*, which show what proportion of the data lies in each of a number of ranges (often called "bins").

Q: What type of data are the following: (a) the height of people in a classroom, (b) the gender of people?

****

(a) Height can be measured on a scale, and so is continuous, while (b) gender is binary.

2.2 Populations and Samples

Statistics is usually concerned about answering a question about a given *population*. A population typically means a well-defined real group of people, or other individual subjects of study, with something in common. For example people who live in the UK, or people aged 65 or over, or even people

2.2. POPULATIONS AND SAMPLES

who enjoy a certain hobby.

Q: Which of the following are populations: (a) People under 18 in Scotland, (b) all cats in Glasgow (c) the centaurs of the world of the Narnia stories by C.S. Lewis?

****

I hope you realised that (a) and (b) are real individuals who can be "units of study", and so form suitable populations, whereas (c) are not, because they are imaginary.[1]

We cannot, however, usually study a whole population, because we don't have the resources. A rare example may be a national census, which tries, as far as possible, to include everybody. Even this cannot include, for example, people who wish to conceal their presence for any reason. So we make do with a *sample*, which we hope is representative of the population. To ensure this, we try to arrange that the each member of the population has an equal chance of being selected - that is, we have a *random* sample.

---

[1] It is true that idealised populations created for the purposes of statistical analysis are also imaginary, but they are related to the real world in a way that mythical creatures are not.

2.3 The Normal distribution

Many biological or psychological measurements[2] follow a mathematical pattern called the "Normal distribution"[3]. A histogram of data that follows this pattern looks like a symmetrical hill when drawn on a graph.

We won't go into the mathematical details of the Normal distribution, but it can be described using the mean of a population and the SD[4]. It has a useful property, which is that about two-thirds[5] of observations fall within one SD of the mean, a range that is 2 SDs long. This can be useful in eliciting the SD if a clinician does not know it, and it is not found in literature.

Q: A clinician who wants a sample size calculation does not know the SD of his observations. However he can say from his experience that a range containing about two-thirds of observations is (95, 135). How can he estimate the SD?

****

The range is 135-95 = 40 units long, which is

---

[2] Measurements that can vary across different individuals e.g. height and weight are called *variables*.

[3] This is partly because they are influenced by many other things, and the total result (especially when they act independently) are liable to follow such a pattern.

[4] which we try to *estimate* from a sample.

[5] 68.3%, to be more precise.

about 2 SDs, so a reasonable estimate would be 20 units. This range would need to be centred about the mean or middle value, of course.

2.4 Samples are not all the same

Although different samples contain different individuals, each sample being only a selection of the whole population, we hope that they are similar in their *group* properties, for example in the proportions of women they contain, or the mean weight of individuals in a sample. In particular, we would also hope that they would be similar to each other in measurements made as part of a scientific study such as a clinical trial, called *outcomes*.

They will not be exactly the same, however. It follows that the mean of a measurement on one sample, for example will not usually be exactly the same as that of the population. As an estimate it may be useful, but it will have some uncertainty. The smaller the sample, the greater the uncertainty (or the less *precise* the finding).

Q: Which of the following will give the most precise estimate of the average height of a population: (a) a sample of 50 people (b) a sample of 100 people (c) a sample of 150 people restricted to men?

****

A sample of 100 people will give a more precise

estimate, but the 150 will not, because it will be selective, and so not representative of the whole population.

2.5 Confidence Intervals

Given our estimate, we express our uncertainty about it by forming a *confidence interval*. For example, if our estimate from our sample is 100 units, we might be able to calculate the confidence interval as (75, 125). This is a plausible range of values for the population value which we cannot measure directly. A larger sample would give us a narrower confidence interval, and so a more precise estimate.

The type of confidence interval used most often is a "95% confidence interval". This means that 95% of such confidence intervals would contain the true value (which makes it reasonable to suppose that ours probably does).

Confidence intervals in clinical trials are often constructed for *differences*, to see if there is evidence for the superiority of a new treatment. To interpret such confidence intervals, we should ask if they contain zero. If they do, that means that we do not have firm evidence of a difference.

Q: Which of the following findings are evidence for a difference in the populations that two arms of a clinical trial come from: (a) sample estimate of the difference 6, confidence interval (-3, 15), (b) sample estimate of the difference 5.5, confidence interval $(4,7)$?

****

Confidence interval (a) contains zero - you can tell because one end is negative and the other is positive. No evidence for a difference. (b) does not contain zero - you can tell because both ends have the same sign (both positive, in this case). We have evidence of a difference.

2.6 Statistical tests

Statistical tests are used to find evidence for something of scientific interest (like a clinically important difference between two groups). To carry them out, we calculate a test statistic from the sample which should (if there is no difference) fall in a certain range. If the value we get is unusual, so that, if there really were no difference, the chance of one as extreme as ours would be very low, we call that "significant" - but note that this is not the same thing as being important in *real* terms, i.e. a *clinically important* difference. This chance, of such a fluke result, is called the "*p*-value", and we want it to be low. The traditional cut-off for statistical significance is 5%.

2.7 Power

If there really is a clinically important difference between two groups (like the arms of a trial), we want to have a good chance of detecting it (which means obtaining a *p*-value under 5%, or a confidence interval for the difference that does *not* contain zero). This chance depends on the sample size and the variability of the measurement, and is the *power*, which should be high. A common traditional cut-off is 80%, but we might choose a higher value like 90%, if we want to be more careful, and resources permit.

2.8 Sample size

In organising a clinical trial, it would be unethical to waste the time of subjects by subjecting them to an experiment which had no hope of answering a question of real interest. Therefore research ethics committees require applicants to provide a scientific justification of their sample size. This means providing information that can be used to show that their study is large enough to have a good chance (*power*) of finding the answer to the question.

Q: Should an ethics committee pass a study that has a power of 50% for detecting a difference that it hopes to find evidence for?

****

The answer is No. The study is, as we say, underpowered *and might well fail to find evidence for an importance difference, even if it were there.*

In that case the time of subjects and public resources would have been wasted.

2.9 Precision

We are not always concerned with proving a difference between two groups. Sometimes we might wish to look at a number that applies only to one group, like a proportion. Here we might do a *precision* calculation, which means having a sample that is large enough to lead to a confidence interval that is narrow enough. The idea of *power* does not apply here.

2.10 Correlation

Correlation is the degree to which the relationship between measurements of two variables on the same individual looks like a straight line when the pairs of measurements for several individuals are plotted on a graph. A positive correlation means that low values of one variable are associated with low values of the other, and similarly for higher values. The symbol r is often used for it when measured from a sample. A value of 1 means that the points fall on a perfect straight line. A value of zero can mean no relationship, as a cloud of points on a graph with no discernable trend would indicate.[6]

---

[6] However a correlation coefficient of zero need not always mean no relationship at all. For example, it may be that the relationship is curved.

Correlations can even be negative, so that low values of one variable are associated with high values of another (and vice versa).

2.11 Prevalence and Incidence

These are two ideas from Epidemiology. They come from Medical research studies which involve simply *observing* individuals (or making use of past observations), not *experimenting* on them with new interventions (which is what clinical trials involve).

Prevalence is a proportion, the fraction of people with a certain condition at one time.

Incidence brings in time or duration more explicitly. Suppose we observe a number of people, say 1000, over a year. That means we have 1000 *person-years* worth of observation. You can see that the idea of "person-years" is similar to "person-hours" or "person-months" in industry. Now we observe how many cases of a condition have occurred over that time. Suppose it is 50. Then the incidence (or incidence *rate*) is 50 cases per 1000 person-years, or 0.05 cases per person-year.

Q: Of 50 people, 3 are found in a survey to have smoked. What is the prevalence of smoking in that group?

****

2.12. RANDOMIZED CLINICAL TRIALS

The prevalence is

$$\frac{3}{50} = 0.06,$$

which is 6%.

Now try this question.

Q: Suppose we observe 10 people over a year and observe 8 cases of a condition. What is the incidence rate per person-year?

****

We have 8 cases per 10 person-years, which is 0.8 cases per person-year.

2.12 Randomized Clinical Trials

Much of this book is written with the organisers of Randomized Clinical Trials (or RCTs) in mind. Such studies are considered the "gold standard" of evidence in Medical Research. They are, in principle, capable of proving that a given intervention *causes* a desired beneficial effect, and is not merely *associated* with it by coincidence.

They typically rely on creating two groups of people that are comparable in every way except for the intervention. This is achieved by *randomly* allocating people to one arm of the trial or the other.

Random allocation is the equivalent of tossing a fair coin, though nowadays it is done by computer.

Though we cannot prove the efficacy of an intervention in the case of an *individual* (because we cannot turn the clock back and ask what would have happened if we had done things differently), an RCT enables us to do so for *groups* of people.

It is by such means that we prove the efficacy of vaccines, for example - by showing that the *risk* of infection is greatly reduced in the experimental arm.

As an example, when Pfizer developed a vaccine for Covid-19, its efficacy was proved by following up two trial arms, till well after the new vaccine would have had time to kick in. One early analysis was carried out when 170 cases of Covid-19 had accumulated.

The result was that 162 of the cases were in the control arm (given a fake substance or *placebo*) while only 8 were found in the experimental arm. Since the trial arms were of near-equal size thanks to the method of allocation, that meant that the risk of Covid had been reduced proportionately from 162 to 8 (or by 95%) in the vaccine arm. That is where the term "95% efficacy" comes from.

Because RCTs are experiments on human beings, strict ethics regulations and laws have been introduced across the world to make sure that the interventions they are designed to test benefit people, and do no harm. Plans for RCTs have to pass scrutiny by Research Ethics Committees or RECs. One of the things they look for is that the sample size is adequate (so that the time and commitment of patients is not wasted, apart from material resources). This book has been written as a help for researchers to that end.

2.13 Diagnostic test studies

In running a diagnostic test, we want to be sure of detecting a condition if someone has it, but also giving them the all-clear if they do not.

Two statistics we often study are the *sensitivity*, which is the proportion of people with the condition for which our test gives a positive result, or "red flag", and the *specificity*, which is the proportion of people who do *not* have the condition, who are given a negative result, or "all-clear".

To find them, however we also need a so-called "gold standard" method of diagnosis, which can diagnose (or clear) people with certainty, against which our new test can be measured. This might not always be a laboratory measurement. An assessment by a senior clinician or other professional may sometimes be the best we can do.

Each of these proportions has their *complement*. If, of 100 people with a condition, a test picks up 90, there are 10 which it fails to pick up, the "false negatives". Thus the *complement* of the sensitivity is the proportion of "false negatives". Again, if we have 100 people without the condition and our test gives the all-clear to 95 of them, that leaves 5 of the 100, or 5% who are "false positives"[7].

---

[7]This fraction is the complement of the *specificity*.

2.14 Epidemiological studies

Very many Epidemiological studies are of two types: *cohort* and *case-control* studies. With cohort or *prospective studies*, we compare a group exposed to some risk factor to another that is not exposed, and follow them up. This can be done in theory with records from the past, making them *historical* cohort studies.

Case-control or *retrospective* studies compare cases of a condition to those who do not have the condition and then enquire about the past, to see which people were exposed (or not) to some risk factor.[8]

Statistical modelling is a common method for analysing such studies and requires the use of statistical software. A statistical model relates an outcome, the *response*, which is often binary (the presence or absence of a condition) to one or more *explanatory variables*. The response is often called "dependent" because it *depends* on the values of the explanatory variables. The explanatory variables are often called "independent".

2.15 Preliminary studies

There are studies where we don't need a power calculation. An example is a preliminary study (often called a *feasibility*, *Phase II* or *pilot*) in which we aim to gather information (such as the SD) that

---

[8]The term *retrospective* may also be used for historical cohort studies, as finding the relevant records involves looking back in time.

2.16. LOOKING AHEAD

will be used later to design a definitive (or *Phase III*) study. A *pilot*, as its name suggests, also has the purpose of uncovering problems that may arise in practice, e.g. with recruitment, or compliance with treatment.

2.16 Looking ahead

You now have enough background for understanding sample size calculations. Subsequent chapters will take you through the common types of sample size calculation, but you will not need advanced Mathematics - a calculator that can do basic arithmetic will be enough.[9]

You may assume that, unless otherwise stated, we will aim for 80% power and a significance level of 5% in our calculations. It is also worth saying that sample size calculations are guidelines rather than rules set in stone, as the assumed figures may often be subjective or approximate.

---

[9]The technical appendix is only for reference, or for statisticians interested in the theoretical background.

Chapter 3

Preliminary studies

3.1 Context

The development of research studies, particularly those related to clinical trials, can be seen as a cycle: initial exploration of the literature, which leads to *preliminary* studies (the subject of this chapter), which are preparatory for *definitive* studies, which lead to Epidemiological studies of the intervention in the wider community or real life, and any long-term side-effects or unintended effects, which in turn lead to new ideas and the planning of new studies from scratch. And so the cycle begins again.

Our main interest here is the second and third of these. It may useful to think of them as building on sound foundations. Good definitive studies build on good preliminary studies, and without good foundations a building is liable to collapse. In the case of clinical trials, that means failure to answer the scientific question. We will say more about this in the section on pilots.

We might think of the foundation itself as having layers: *safety and efficacy* (or dose-finding studies), *feasibility* studies, and *pilots*, though the latter two are not always separated. As will be seen below, we might regard pilots as a special class of feasibility studies.

3.2 Dose finding studies

We don't deal here in detail with modern methods for dose finding studies that use statistical modelling, which is a specialised topic in itself. However it is worth mentioning a simple time-honoured method, the so-called "3+3"[1]. We use a succession of cohorts of three subjects given increasing doses of a drug. The first dose is intentionally very low, e.g. one tenth of a dose that would kill one tenth of mice.

The increase is a proportion of the previous dose, and this decreases each time up to a point. One possible sequence of such proportional increases might be 100% (second dose double the first), 67%, 50% (fourth dose half as much again as the third), and 33% thereafter.

The dose is increased until people start to report undesirable side effects. If only one patient reports side effects, we may try with another cohort at the same dose (though a third chance will not be given). If two experience side-effects out of three, we stop

---

[1]Further details of this and other designs will be found in Storer (1989).

and use the highest dose that was tolerated by all three.[2] For this sort of experiment, 20-30 in total should be sufficient.

The above method is used to find the maximum *tolerated* dose, and is done on *healthy* volunteers.

However we also need to find an *effective* dose, and this can be done by testing the drug in different doses on people who actually need treatment, but this time restricting the doses used to a range that we know to be safe.

3.3 Feasibility studies

It is important to note what feasibility studies are *not* designed to do. Being preliminary studies, they are not intended to provide definitive evidence - that comes from the next stage. For this reason they do not aim to satisfy power calculations. Their aim is rather to provide information that will help design definitive studies. They should give us some idea of the differences we might expect to see across the arms in the main outcome measurements, and the variability of those measurements.

Even such studies assume, however, that safety and efficacy studies have already been carried out. The latter may be regarded as the lowest part of the 'foundations' that we referred to earlier. The information that we need for planning a definitive study, that we are most likely to get from a feasi-

---

[2]In soccer terminology, one reported side effect would merit a 'yellow card', but two (or indeed two yellow cards in succession) would merit a 'red card'.

bility study, is an estimate of the SD of the main outcome, or of the likely proportions in each arm, in the case of binary outcomes. This will give us some idea of the variability in the data.

There is no one ideal sample size for doing this, but a typical figure[3] is 30 per arm for continuous outcomes, and so we suggest such a size. For trials involving proportions, however the numbers required in a definitive trial are liable to be higher, and so, if resources permit, a higher figure like 50 per arm for feasibility studies may be desirable.

3.4 Pilot studies

We might be tempted to think of preliminary studies as being mainly feasibility studies. However we can distinguish pilots as having a distinct function of their own.[4] It is to act as *scale models*, revealing problems that are liable to arise in practice. Such information can be just as vital as the information gained from feasibility studies about the main outcome measurement.

A study may fail to answer a scientific question because of deficiencies in recruitment, compliance with treatment or the quality of collected data. The first two of these can mean that the study is underpowered because of lack of numbers. if we find out too late, that either the recruitment rate or com-

---

[3]See, for example Totton, Lin, Julious, Chowdhury, and Brand (2023).

[4]For this reason we treat them separately, though they could be thought of as a special case of feasibility studies.

3.4. PILOT STUDIES

pliance with the intervention is not what we hoped it would be, our study may fail to gather enough evidence to effectively answer our question. Data in the form of numbers and codes should be ideally recorded in a standard form, and not in text fields that leave interpretation to chance. If the quality of collected data is not good, we may not be able to gain any useful information from it by analysis.

It should be clear from the above that pilots are just as vital as feasibility studies, though both may be combined in the same project.

Potential sponsors, or members of funding committees may indeed wish to be satisfied about the quality of preliminary studies, or relevant evidence from them, before approving grants for larger definitive studies, to avoid a large waste of money and other resources, not least the time of patients and families.

Q: How large should the size of a pilot be, for a continuous outcome?

****

The sample size for a pilot study as such is not a fixed number - it is any number large enough to bring out problems in practice. However if a feasibility study also serves as a pilot, then 30 per arm should be a suitable number.

Chapter 4

Two arms

4.1 Types of outcome

Imagine a randomized clinical trial with two arms. To calculate a sample size, you need a clearly defined and measurable outcome. This may be a continuous measurement, or a binary outcome (Yes/No). In general, trials with binary outcomes are larger, because more information is available from continuous measurements.

Q: Consider two trials, in which the first has systolic blood pressure as the outcome, while in the second, the outcome is the occurrence (or not) of vomiting. Which is likely to be larger?

****

Blood pressure is a continuous measure (mmHg). The presence of vomiting is a binary outcome. So the second trial is liable to be larger. Note that blood pressure could be made into a binary measure by regarding hypertension (e.g systolic blood pressure over 140) as the outcome. This would lead to a loss of information, and the resulting trial would need to be larger.

4.2 Caution about assuming Normality

We are going to assume that continuous outcomes are Normally distributed. However, in practice you may come up against observations which are not Normally distributed. For example they may have a constraint imposed on them. An example would be observations which might have a Normal distribution, but which for a particular study are only accepted if they are above a threshold. That creates a *truncated* distribution to which our methods wouldn't apply, and it would be necessary to see a statistician for further help in that case. The same would apply to outcomes which needed to be transformed before their distribution became reasonably close to Normal[1]. If in doubt, see a statistician.

---

[1] Two common ways are taking logs (to the base e), and square root. If it works, a histogram of the transformed data should look roughly like a symmetrical hill.

4.3 Continuous Outcomes

We now come to a basic principle. The sample size depends critically on how the size of the clinically important difference, if known (which we will abbreviate to CID) in an outcome compares to the size of the SD. Take note of the following fact, because we will use it as a point of departure:

Given the aim of 80% power and 5% significance, if the CID is the same as the SD, we need 16 people per arm.

Now if the SD is bigger relative to the CID, the required sample size will be bigger. How much bigger? If the SD is doubled, we will need *four* times as many subjects.

Q: If the CID is 5 units and the SD is 10 units, how many people will we need per arm?

****

Since the SD is twice that of the CID, we will need 4×16, i.e. 64 per arm.

This should give you an idea of how to calculate sample size. Divide the SD by the CID, and *square* the result. Then multiply by 16, and you have the sample size. For example, suppose the CID is 20 and the SD is 36. The ratio of SD to CID is 1.8, and its square is 3.24. 3.24×16 is 51.84. Rounding up, you will need 52 per group.

Now try this example.

Q: Suppose the CID is 5 units and the SD is 6 units. how many people will you need per arm?

****

The ratio of SD to CID is 1.2, and its square is 1.44. 1.44 × 16 is 23.04. So you should manage comfortably if you recruit 24 per group. You may get away with 23 per group, though the power would be slightly short of 80%, but I would play safe, unless you have difficulty getting the number, and the project is important.

You may ask what you should do if the power you want is 90% instead of 80%. In that case you use 21 where you have used 16 above. Try this question based on the example above, which needed 64 per arm for 80% power.

Q: If the CID is 5 units and the SD is 10 units, how many people will we need per arm to get 90% power?

****

Since the SD is twice that of the CID, we will need 4× 21, i.e. 84 per group.

4.4 Proportions

To calculate a sample size using proportions, you need to know the expected proportion with the binary outcome in both arms, control and experimental. The calculations would require complex formulae, so to save you the trouble I have provided a table which will enable you to calculate the sample size for the ones you are likely to use most frequently. The order of the arms does not matter. Note that the proportions p_1 and p_2 here are *percentages*.

You will see that the sample size (the number required per arm) is the same whether the expected proportions in the arms (expressed here as % ages) are p_1 and p_2 or their respective complements $(100 - p_1)$ and $(100 - p_2)$. For completeness, numbers are given for 90% power as well as 80%. You will see that the assumed clinically important difference is either 10% or 5%. Though these are round numbers, remember that *this is not a statistical question*. What is important in real terms is something that *you* may well be the best judge of.

The figures in the table are rounded *up* to the nearest integer, except where the first digit after the decimal point was zero. Then they're rounded down.[2]

Now here are two questions for practice, which require you to use the table.

---

[2] We follow this policy in tables generally, where sample sizes are calculated to the nearest integer, as in Chapter 6.

p_1	p_2		p_1	p_2	80%	90%
5	10	=	90	95	424	568
10	15	=	85	90	681	911
10	20	=	80	90	195	261
15	20	=	80	85	903	1208
15	25	=	75	85	248	332
20	30	=	70	80	292	391
30	40	=	60	70	356	476
40	50	=	50	60	388	519

Table 4.1: Sample sizes for proportions.

Q: The control proportion in one arm of a trial of an undesirable binary outcome is 50%, and we hope for a proportion of 40% in the experimental arm. What number do we need to recruit per arm to pick up such a difference with 80% power?

****

You need 380 per arm. See the last line of the table, and see the first pair of values. Remember that the order doesn't matter.

Now try this one.

Q: Same question as above, but now we aim for 90% power. How many do we need?

4.4. PROPORTIONS

****

You need 519 per arm.

4.4.1 Proportions not in the table

You may well ask "What if the proportions I expect or hope are not in the table you've provided?" The following method will give you a good approximate answer. Recall that in dealing with continuous outcomes, you calculate a multiplier, which inflates the basic sample sizes of 16 per group (for 80% power) or 21 (for 90% power). To calculate the multiplier here, you need the expected proportions p_1 and p_2. You then calculate their average $\bar{p}$. The multiplier you need is then

$$\frac{\bar{p}(1-\bar{p})}{(p_1-p_2)^2}.$$

Here's an example. Suppose the expected proportions are $p_1 = 0.4$ and $p_2 = 0.6$. Then their average is

$$\bar{p} = \frac{0.4 + 0.6}{2} = 0.5.$$

Its complement $(1 - \bar{p}) = 1 - 0.5 = 0.5$, and so the multiplier is

$$\frac{0.5 \times 0.5}{(0.4 - 0.6)^2} = \frac{0.25}{0.04} = 6.25.$$

So (for 80% power) we multiply 16 by 6.25, giving 100 per arm.

Q: Suppose the expected proportions are 0.7 and 0.9. For 80% power, how many will you need per arm?

****

Here the expected proportions are $p_1 = 0.7$ and $p_2 = 0.9$. So their average is

$$\bar{p} = \frac{0.7 + 0.9}{2} = 0.8.$$

Its complement $(1 - \bar{p}) = 1 - 0.8 = 0.2$, and so the multiplier is

$$\frac{0.8 \times 0.2}{(0.7 - 0.9)^2} = \frac{0.16}{0.04} = 4.$$

So (for 80% power) we multiply 16 by 4, giving 64 per arm.

Now try this question.

Q: Suppose we wished to pick up this difference with 90% power. What would be the sample size?

****

You would multiply 21 by the multiplier, giving 84 per arm.

4.4.2 Survival studies

Many "survival" studies are concerned with the time to an undesirable event, such as the recurrence

4.5. ALLOWING FOR DROPOUTS

of a serious illness, or a vascular incident. We can apply the methods for proportions if the outcome is expressed as the proportion of people surviving a certain period. For example in some cancer studies the main outcome of interest may be a remission lasting for 5 years, and so the "5-year survival" is the proportion of people who have so survived. Shorter periods such as two years or even less might be used for more serious illnesses.

4.5 Allowing for dropouts

We cannot always assume that the numbers we have aimed to recruit will be achieved in the time set for a study. People may opt out, or drop out for a number of reasons.[3] We can allow for this by increasing the number by an appropriate amount. Think about this question.

Q: Suppose you need 64 for each arm of a trial, and you have reason to believe that half will drop out. How many should you try to recruit?

****

I hope you saw that you will need to double *your numbers to 128 per arm, so that even if half dropped out, you would be left with 64 per arm.*

---

[3]Note that this is not a failure to take treatment, i.e. of *compliance*. We deal with this in the chapter on Optional topics.

Often however matters may not be so simple. To deal with any proportion p of dropouts, you first need to express it as a number between 0 and 1 (not as a percentage). Thus if the proportion of dropouts is 25%, p is 0.25.

Q: Suppose you have reason to believe that 27% will drop out. What will p be?

****

Here p is
$$\frac{27}{100} = 0.27.$$

You then need to follow this rule:

If the proportion dropping out is p, divide the sample size by $(1 - p)$.

Remember that p here is a proportion between 0 and 1, not a percentage. So if the expected dropout rate were 25%, p would be 0.25, and you would divide by 0.75. You can do this with a simple calculator.

Now try this example.

Q: Suppose you need 128 for each arm of a trial, and you have reason to believe that 20% will drop out. How many should you try to recruit?

****

4.6. HEDGING YOUR BETS

Here p is 0.2, and $(1 - p)$ is 0.8, so you need to divide 128 by 0.8 which you can do with a simple calculator. The result is 160, which you need to aim to recruit.

It is a good idea to round *upwards* to a suitable round number when applying this method, as the next section will show.

4.6 Hedging your bets

There are a number of ways of doing sample size calculations, and they give similar results, but not exactly the same. Some books (including ours) use approximate methods which are easy to use with a calculator.[4] Here are some ways of allowing for this.

To begin with, always round your sample size calculation *upwards*, not downwards. Then, *if your calculated sample size before rounding is below 41, and rounding up means an increase of less than half a unit, increase it by 1 after rounding up*. The result should be no less than numbers obtained with more sophisticated methods.

Q: Suppose your clinically important difference is 5, and the SD is 8. For proving this CID with 80% power, 5% significance, what number should you aim at?

---

[4]One approximate (but good) method uses a graph called Altman's nomogram, which we will not deal with here. You will find further details in Altman (1991).

****

The ratio of SD to CID is 1.6, whose square is 2.56. Multiplying this by 16 (for 80% power) gives 40.96. Rounding upwards gives 41, which is an increase of only 0.05. So increasing by 1, we get the answer, 42.

Now try this question.

Q: In an earlier example the clinically important difference was 5, and the SD was 6. Would our answer need increasing by 1?

****

In that example the answer was 23.04, and rounding up to 24 would mean an increase of more than 0.5. Therefore we would not *need to increase the answer beyond 24.*

You may in fact not need the unit increase at all, if you increase your recruitment figures to allow for dropouts. This should also iron out the (small) differences between different methods for finding sample sizes. If you do this, since drop out estimates are liable to be only rough, I suggest that you choose a round number to aim at for recruitment. For example, if you need to recruit between 75 and 80, and you expect about 1 in 6, or between 15% and 20% to drop out, you could aim to recruit 100 - to allow both for dropouts *and* the small differences in methods for calculating sample sizes.

Q: *Suppose your calculations (after rounding up) say that you need 36 for each arm of a trial. What might you do if (a) you do not expect anyone to drop out, (b) you expect up to 15% to drop out?*

****

(a) You could add 1 to 36 and so aim to recruit 37 per arm. (b) Dividing 36 by the complement of 15% which is 0.85, you get 42.4, and rounding upwards to a suitable round number, you could aim to recruit 45 or even 50 per arm.

4.7 Research Ethics committees

In many countries, if you are planning a trial you will need to go through a REC or Research Ethics Committee. This is a panel of a mixture of experts, which often has a Statistical advisor. If you are planning a definitive study, you will need to provide enough information to enable them to check that your sample size is sufficiently large. You may assume that the required significance level of any statistical test is 5% and that the minimum power to be aimed at is 80%. In addition, for continuous outcomes, you will need to provide the clinically important difference (which is *not* a statistical question) that you hope to find evidence for, and also the variability (SD) of the primary outcome measurement. As we said earlier, if you don't have this information to hand or in literature, you may base it on clinical experience, assuming that the outcome is even approximately Normally distributed: a range of values containing about two-thirds of likely values covers two SDs, so half of this is a suitable estimate.

For trials of proportions, you will also need to supply two pieces of information, but they are different: you will need the expected proportion in the control arm, *and* the expected proportion in the experimental arm.

The above applies to *superiority trials*. For *non-inferiority trials*, for continuous outcomes, instead of the clinically important difference you supply the *tolerance* - the extent to which the lower limit of the confidence interval for the "advantage" of the experimental intervention can be allowed to go below zero (and it mustn't do so further than a clinically important amount). For proportions, you supply the tolerance instead of the expected proportion in the experimental arm. Again, it mustn't exceed a clinically important amount.

Chapter 5

Precision

Precision calculations are usually done for *proportions*. If an estimate of a proportion from a sample is 50%, and the confidence interval is (40%, 60%) the precision is 10%. We do not want the ends of a confidence interval to be too far from our estimate for a proportion. But how far is too far is not a statistical question. A precision of 10% might be good enough for some purposes, but others may require a finer estimate.

Q: For the estimate of 50%, suppose we want a precision of 5%. What should the confidence interval look like?

****

The confidence interval should be contained in the interval (45%, 55%) as tightly as possible, so that the ends of the interval are no more than 5% from

Estimate		Precision	
p_1	p_2	5%	10%
10	90	200	70
15	85	260	80
20	80	300	85
25	75	324	92
30	70	350	100
35	65	380	100
40	60	380	100
45	55	400	100
	50	400	100

Table 5.1: Sample sizes for precision

the estimate - but at the same time, the interval should not be narrower than is necessary.

We now come to the question of big our sample needs to be. This depends on two things: the expected proportion, and the precision. Again, any formula to calculate this would not be simple, and so I have provided a table to enable you to do this for common cases. I have provided the size of sample you would need for a precision of 5% and 10% for estimated proportions between 10% and 90%. The symbols p_1 and p_2 indicate complementary proportions (which add to 100%), and mean that for both proportions the required numbers are the same. The complement of 50% is itself, so only one proportion is needed in the last line of the table. Please note that estimating extreme proportions such as 5% (or its complement) 95%, or more extreme ones, is very difficult, and only possible in very large and expensive studies. Therefore I have not tried to go further then 10% or 90%. Here's an exercise to give you a little practice in using the table.

Q: How big should your sample be, if you want to estimate (a) a proportion of 70% with a precision of 10%, (b) a proportion of 25% with a precision of 5%? What will the answers be for their complements, i.e. 30% in the case of (a) and 75% in the case of (b)?

****

The answers are (a) 100, (b) 324. Note that the answers will be the same for the complements of the estimated proportions, so that to estimate a proportion 30% with a precision of 10% we will need a sample of size 100, while to estimate one of 75% with a precision of 5%, we will need a sample of size 324.

One thing you should be aware of, though a technical matter, is that more precise "Wilson" confidence intervals for proportions (except 50%) are not symmetrical. In calculating sample sizes, we have chosen to err on the side of caution, and so the precision is that of the *narrower* arm of the interval.

Chapter 6

Optional topics

This chapter contains topics rather harder than the earlier part of the book. You may consider them as optional, unless of course you intend to use them in your work.

6.1 Multiple testing

If two primary outcomes are being studied, we can allow for the possibility of fluke results by tightening the significance level from 5% to 2.5%. This involves increasing the sample size by a percentage. For 80% power this is 21%, while for 90% power it is 18%.[1] If you use 20% as an approximation, however, you won't go far wrong, provided you have already marked the size up to allow for dropouts.

---

[1] This may seem counter-intuitive, but we are talking about the difference that multiple testing makes, not added power.

Q: A sample size for 80% power, 5% is 100 per arm. You decide to measure two outcomes which are similar and so lower the significance level to 2.5%. What will the new sample size be?

****

An increase of 21% will make it 121 per arm. As I have said, however, if you had arrived at 100 after allowing for dropouts, you wouldn't go far wrong by aiming for 120, and that would be adequate.

6.2 Unequal arms

Sometimes you may have more people available for one arm of a trial than the other. How do you modify the sample size to allow for this? We will begin by assuming that the ratio of the size of arm A to that of arm B is r. Thus if $r = 2$, arm A has twice as many people as arm B. Note that A and B may refer respectively to the control and the experimental arm in either order. Then we proceed as follows:

1. Suppose the size of the arms, had they been equal, would have been $2k$. For example, if the size of each arm was 16, k would be 8.

2. Then the size of arm A will be $(r+1)k$, while that of arm B will be

$$\left(\frac{r+1}{r}\right)k.$$

For both arms we multiply the expression involving r by k. In this case $r + 1 = 2+1 = 3$, so that the

6.2. UNEQUAL ARMS

size of arm A is $3 \times 8 = 24$. As for arm B,

$$\left(\frac{r+1}{r}\right) = \left(\frac{2+1}{2}\right) = 1.5.$$

So the size of arm B is $1.5 \times 8 = 12$. Now try this example.

Q: A trial with equal arms would have 120 per arm. Not sure that you will be able to recruit that many, you hope to make one arm 3 times as bigger than the other in the hope that the smaller arm will not need as many. How many can you save?

****

Here

$$k = \frac{120}{2} = 60.$$

$r = 3$, *so the larger arm has* $(3+1) \times 60 = 240$. *For the smaller arm,*

$$\left(\frac{r+1}{r}\right) = \left(\frac{3+1}{3}\right) = \frac{4}{3}.$$

So the size of arm B is

$$\frac{4}{3} \times 60 = 80.$$

Thus you would save recruiting 40 in the smaller arm.

6.3 Compliance

If a proportion p of patients are expected to fail to take their treatment this is a more serious problem than simple dropout, because it affects the treatment effect that we can hope to find. To allow for it we need to divide the size of each arm n by $(1-p)^2$, i.e. the *square* of the complement of p. For example, if our basic sample size is 100, and we expect that 10% will drop out, then $p = 0.1$, so $(1-p)^2 = 0.81$ and so the size of each arm n is

$$\frac{100}{0.81} = 123.5,$$

and rounding up we need to recruit 124 per arm.

Q: Suppose your expected size is 80, but you expect half the recruits to not take treatment. How many will you need to recruit per arm?

****

Here $p = 0.5$, so its complement is 0.5. So we divide by $0.5^2 = 0.25$. So the size of each arm n is

$$\frac{80}{0.25} = 320.$$

You can see that sample size is sensitive to failure of compliance in the same way as the SD.

6.3.1 A note on analysis

This book doesn't deal with the analysis of results, but we will say here that a failure of compliance dilutes the effect of an intervention, and we can allow for it by dividing the treatment effect by the compliance, i.e. by $(1-p)$. This is the *Complier-Averaged* effect, but to establish its validity we would need to show that the "compliers" (people taking their treatment) were demographically similar to the rest of the treatment arm.

Q: Suppose 25% of people in a treatment arm do not take it. How would you allow for this in analysis?

****

Here $p = 0.25$ and its complement is 0.75. So you would divide the treatment effect by 0.75, effectively increasing it by a third.

6.3.2 A note on policy

Allowing for failure of compliance may tell us how well the treatment would work under ideal conditions, but in the real worlld we may be more concerned about the effect of the policy of the treatment, and so unless we find a way of improving compliance, the complier-averaged effect will have only academic value.

6.4 Clusters

Sometimes the units of study are not individuals but *groups*, where individuals are related to each other in some way: households, classrooms or even general practices. This means that the measurements are not independent, and consequently we need to multiply the sample size by an *inflation factor*. This involves knowledge of a statistic that measures clustering which is not easy to obtain, called the ICC (intra cluster correlation). If you obtain it, however[2] and have the cluster size m as well as the ICC which we will call c, the inflation factor is $1 + (m-1)c$.

Q: If the ICC is 0.05 and the size of the cluster is 25, what is the inflation factor? If the sample size without clustering would have been 100 per arm, how many clusters will be required (rounded up)?

****

Here $m = 25$ and $c = 0.05$, so the inflation factor is $1 + (25-1) \times 0.05 = 1 + 1.20 = 2.20$. Hence the size of each arm without clustering, 100, is multiplied by 2.2, making 220 people per arm. To find the number of clusters we divide the total number per arm by the cluster size.

$$\frac{220}{25} = 8.8.$$

Rounding up we will need 9 clusters per arm.

Further details about cluster trials will be found in Eldridge and Kerry (2012).

---

[2] A commonly assumed value for clinical trials might be 0.05 or 5%, but possible assumed or reported values could range from 0.01 or 1%, to 0.1 or 10%.

6.5 Rule of 3 for rare events

You may sometimes want to design a study in which you expect rare events. Assume you get 100 observations without a single event. What is the confidence interval for the proportion of rare events? The lower limit *is* zero (since it is zero in your sample), but what about the upper limit? This is

$$\frac{3}{100} = 0.03.$$

So the confidence interval is (0, 0.03).

In general, if you have a sample of size n with *no* events, the upper limit of the confidence interval for the proportion of rare events is

$$\frac{3}{n}.$$

Q: If you have 300 observations with not a single event, what will be the upper limit for the confidence interval for the proportion of rare events?

****

Here the upper limit is

$$\frac{3}{300} = 0.01.$$

So the confidence interval is (0, 0.01).

Suppose now that you want to study a rare event and want the upper limit of the confidence interval to be no more than 5%. Then we have

$$\frac{3}{n} = 0.05.$$

So

$$n = \frac{3}{0.05} = 60.$$

So we will need a run of 60 observations with *no* events, to obtain a confidence interval of (0%, 5%).

Q: Suppose you want the upper limit of the confidence interval to be no more than 4%. How many observations will you need to have without a single event?

****

Here we have

$$\frac{3}{n} = 0.04.$$

So

$$n = \frac{3}{0.04} = 75.$$

So we will need a run of 75 observations with no events, to obtain a confidence interval of (0%, 4%).

6.5.1 Application to Diagnostic Tests

With diagnostic tests, we may wish to measure a proportion, sensitivity or specificity, that is as high

6.5. RULE OF 3 FOR RARE EVENTS

as possible. But estimating extreme proportions is very difficult. To measure a proportion of 95%, for example, with a precision of 1%, we would need a sample of size 2200, and even then the lower limit of the confidence interval would be 94%.

However there is a more economical solution that exploits the "Rule of 3". Suppose we want the lower limit of the confidence interval for the specificity to be at least 95%. Then the proportion of people without the condition who are given a *false* positive result will have to have an upper confidence limit of 5%. The Rule of 3 tells us that to do this we will need a run of

$$\frac{3}{0.05} = 60.$$

Thus if we get a straight run of 60 people who are normal (according to a gold standard) with no false positive results, we can conclude that the confidence interval for false positives is (0%, 5%), and hence the confidence interval for the specificity is (95%, 100%).

Q: Suppose you want the lower limit for the sensitivity of a diagnostic test to be at least 99%. How many people with a gold standard diagnosis of having the illness will you need to test with no false negative test results to be sure?

****

You need the upper confidence limit for the

proportion of people with the condition whom the test fails to pick up, i.e. false negatives, to be 0.01. By the Rule of 3 you need

$$\frac{3}{0.01} = 300.$$

You will need a straight run of 300 people with the condition, none of whom the test fails to pick up.

6.6 Rule of 10 for Epidemiology

Suppose you wish to find evidence for the relationship between the occurrence of a condition and the exposure (or not) of an individual to one of several possible risk factors. How big should your sample be, in order for you to have a good chance of finding it? There is no one method of power calculation for such questions, because statistical models can be so varied. However among Statisticians there is a well-known 'rule of thumb'[3] which is: *find 10 Yeses and 10 Nos for each explanatory variable you wish to examine.*

In cohort studies, that means finding 10 people exposed and 10 unexposed, for each risk factor you hope to examine. In case-control studies, that means 10 people with a condition and 10 without, for each risk factor. Now try these two questions.

---

[3] Further examples of 'rules of thumb' used in Statistics will be found in van Belle (2008).

6.6. RULE OF 10 FOR EPIDEMIOLOGY

Q: In a cohort study looking at the relationship between smoking status and hypertension as risk factors (both treated as binary conditions), and their influence on the development of lung cancer, leaving aside people with both, how many people will you need to recruit?

****

You will need 10 people who smoke and 10 who don't, and also 10 who have hypertension and 10 who don't, or a minimum of 40.[4]

Now try this one.

Q: You wish to look at risk factors related to a condition, and you can recruit 60 people with the condition and match them with 60 who do not have it. How many possible risk factors might you hope to find evidence for?

****

The rule tells us that you can hope to find evidence for perhaps six risk factors.

The "Rule of 10" is not set in stone, and some people would say that 20 would be even better. That is true in the sense that the more evidence you have, the better. But the rule of 10 may be

---

[4]You might, of course, save a small number if some fall in both categories, but see the caution at the end of the section.

a good guide in planning studies, especially if resources are limited.

6.7 Before-after correlation

Some studies use people as their own controls. This has the advantage of not needing a second comparator group, but it also reduces the sample size required, because there is often a correlation between the first and second observations, which would otherwise be regarded as if they came from two independent groups, like two different trial arms. As it happens, if the expected correlation is r, we can reduce the sample size by multiplying the sample size by $1 - r^2$.

As an example, if the sample size we might have needed is 100, and the correlation is 0.4, the square of 0.4 is 0.16 and $(1 - 0.16) = 0.84$. So we multiply the sample size by 0.84, or 84%, which means a 16% reduction.

Q: Suppose the correlation is 0.5. How much will the sample size be reduced by?

****

Here $r = 0.5$, so $r^2 = 0.25$. $1 - 0.25 = 0.75$, or 75%, which means a 25% reduction.

Note that before-after studies are not a substitute for RCTs, as the effect of *time* comes into them, as well as any intervention.

6.8 Incidence rates

In a trial comparing the incidence across two arms, the sample size depends on the *difference* between the rates, which we hope to pick up. It also depends on the units used. I will provide a basic table and then show you how to alter the figures for different units. The first two columns are observations per person-time unit, while the third column is the number of person-time units of observation that are needed in each arm for detecting the difference with 80% power, and the fourth has the figures for 90% power.

To use the table, you need to convert the control incidence rate to 1 case per person-time unit. Thus 10 cases per 100 person-years will become 1 case per 10 person-years, and so the unit will be 10 person-years. The study arm's incidence rate must also be expressed in terms of this unit, which should yield a number in the second column of the table (assuming of course that your intervention is expected to *reduce* the incidence). The third and fourth column will then tell you how many units you need to obtain.

Here's an example. Suppose you want to compare two arms, where the control has an incidence of 100 cases per 1000 person-years. That is equivalent to 1 case per 10 person-years, so the unit is 10 person-years. Suppose you expect that the experimental or study arm will have an incidence of 50 cases per 1000 person years. That is 0.5 cases per 10 person-years. From the table, you will need 47 of these units per arm to pick up such a difference

Control rate	Study rate	Person-time units/arm (80% power)	Person-time units/arm (90% power)
1	0.05	10	13
1	0.10	11	15
1	0.15	13	17
1	0.20	15	20
1	0.25	18	24
1	0.30	21	28
1	0.35	25	34
1	0.40	31	41
1	0.45	38	51
1	0.50	47	63
1	0.55	60	81
1	0.60	79	105
1	0.65	106	142
1	0.70	149	199
1	0.75	220	295
1	0.80	354	473
1	0.85	646	864
1	0.90	1492	1997
1	0.95	6123	8196

Table 6.1: Sample sizes for rates.

6.8. INCIDENCE RATES

with 80% power, which is 470 person-years. You will need to follow 470 people in each arm over a year (or 235 for each arm over two years etc) to pick up the difference.

Q: Suppose you want to compare two arms where the control has an incidence of 50 cases per 100 person-years and you expect that the control has an incidence of 30 cases per 100 person-years, and you want your investigation to pick up the difference with 90% power. You have two years to complete the study. How many people will you need to recruit in each arm?

****

50 cases per 100 person-years is 1 case per 2 person-years, so your unit is 2 person-years. 30 cases per 100 person-years is $\frac{30}{50} = 0.6$ cases per 2 person-years. From the table, you will need 105 units per arm, that is 210 person-years. You will need to recruit 105 people in each arm for two years.

The above calculation hasn't allowed for dropouts. We'll do that with the next question.

Q: Suppose that you expect a dropout rate of 25%. How will that affect your answer?

****

You will need to divide 105 by (1-0.25) = 0.75, giving 140 people to be aimed at per arm per year.

6.9 Non-inferiority trials

Sometimes a clinical trial doesn't aim at showing that a new treatment is better than an old one by an amount that matters in real terms (the CID). If a new treatment is simply cheaper, or avoids unpleasant side-effects, we may simply wish to show that it is *no worse* than the current one. To do this we specify an acceptable *tolerance*. Given a confidence interval for the "advantage" of the new treatment, the lower end may be allowed to dip below zero, but only by a degree that is not clinically important. Thus the size of this tolerance, like the CID, is *not* a statistical question. That is sufficient to prove "non-inferiority".[5]

6.9.1 Continuous outcomes

The sample size calculation requires us to specify an SD, and a tolerance. We will assume for now that the significance level is 5% and the power 80%. The starting point is similar to that of superiority trials:

Given the aim of 80% power and 5% significance, if the tolerance is the same as the SD, we need 16

---

[5]From the point of *credibility*, however it would be also be good for the estimate of the "advantage" of the experimental treatment, and certainly the *upper* end of the confidence interval, to not be below zero.

6.9. NON-INFERIORITY TRIALS

people per arm.
If they are not the same, we apply a similar principle to superiority trials: we square the ratio of the SD to the tolerance and multiply by 16.

Q: If the tolerance is 10 units and the SD is 20 units, how many people will we need per arm?

****

Since the SD is twice that of the tolerance, we will need 4×16, i.e. 64 per group.

As with superiority trials, if you want 90% power, use a basic figure of 21 instead of 16.

6.9.2 Proportions

For non-inferiority trials using proportions, you need the proportion in the control arm and the acceptable tolerance. In the table that follows, we call these respectively p_C and τ. We assume a tolerance of 10% in the first two columns, and 5% in the third and fourth. For the given control proportions, we have provided the sample sizes for powers of 80% and 90%. The proportions are given as percentages. It is not possible to calculate a sample size where the tolerance equals the control proportion[6], so these cells are blank.

---

[6] As the tolerance gets very close to 10%, the sample size becomes impossibly high.

p_C	τ 10% 80%	τ 10% 90%	τ 5% 80%	τ 5% 90%
95	140	202	392	558
90	178	253	579	815
85	214	302	746	1044
80	245	344	889	1240
75	270	378	1007	1403
70	289	403	1102	1532
65	303	421	1171	1627
60	310	430	1217	1687
55	311	430	1237	1714
50	305	422	1233	1707
45	294	405	1204	1665
40	277	381	1150	1589
35	253	347	1072	1479
30	224	305	969	1335
25	188	255	842	1157
20	147	197	691	945
15	102	133	515	700
10			317	424

Table 6.2: Sample sizes for proportions (non-inferiority).

6.10. FACTORIAL TRIALS

Q: A non-inferiority trial has a control proportion of 80% and a tolerance of 10%. For 90% power, how many people will you need to recruit per arm?

****

From the table you will need 344 per arm.

6.10 Factorial trials

On occasion we may wish to study the effects of two treatments at once. We may wish to know how they act independently, but also whether their effect when they act together is different from the mere sum of their independent effects: in other words, their *interaction*. This requires a trial with four arms, one control, two experimental arms with each of the two treatments alone, and one experimental arm with both treatments acting at once.

Suppose the respective sizes of the outcome measure in the arms is as follows:
Control: A
One of the treatments: B,
Other treatment: C
Both treatments: D
The interaction term is a difference of two differences:
$(A - B) - (C - D)$
which is $A - B - C + D$. Let us called this term I, the interaction term.

To find the sample size, if we can assume that the SD is the same across all four arms, then if the

64   CHAPTER 6. OPTIONAL TOPICS

size of the SD is the same as I, to detect it with 80% power and a significance level of 5% we need 32 per arm. For 90% we would need 42 per arm. If the SD is different, we apply a similar principle to earlier: *square* the ratio of the SD to I, and multiply this by 32 (to detect the interaction with 80% power) or 42 for 90%.

Q: A factorial term has an interaction term of 3 and the SD of all measurements is 6. To detect the interaction with 90% power how large should each arm be?

****

The ratio of the SD to I is 2. So we multiply the square of 2, which is 4, by 42 (for 90% power), giving 168 per arm.

It is possible to organise trials which are still more complex, involving interaction between three or more treatments. We should note, however that the size of an interaction may well be small in magnitude and therefore harder to detect, even if it is (roughly) known in advance. Consequently, such trials are liable to be very expensive, as well as risking a lack of power for detecting the interaction. For this reason, it may be best to avoid them, unless the question of how one treatment influences another when both are present is of vital importance.

Chapter 7

Revision Exercises

This chapter is intended for you, if you have worked through the previous chapters, to test your understanding of the material, and give you further practice.

7.1 Main topics

7.1.1 Two-arm trial: Continuous outcome

Q: The clinical important difference in a trial is 4 units and the SD is 6 units. The expected dropout rate is 10%. How many people will you need per arm for 90% power?

****

For 90% power, if the ratio of SD to CID were 1, the base figure is 21. The ratio of SD to CID is

66   CHAPTER 7. REVISION EXERCISES

1.5, and its square is 2.25. 2.25 × 21 is 47.25. To allow for 10% dropout we need to divide this by (1-0.1) = 0.9, giving 52.5. Rounding up, you should aim for a minimum of 53 per group.

7.1.2   Two-arm trial: Proportions

Q: The control proportion in one arm of a trial of an undesirable binary outcome is 25% and we hope for a proportion of 15% in the experimental arm. What number will you need to recruit per arm to pick up such a difference with 90% power?

****

Using the table, you will need 332 per arm.

Now try this one.

Q: Suppose the expected proportions were 0.65 and 0.5. For 90% power, how many will you need per arm ?

****

Here the expected proportions are $p_1 = 0.65$ and $p_2 = 0.5$. So their average is

$$\bar{p} = \frac{0.65 + 0.0.5}{2} = 0.575.$$

Its complement is

$$(1 - \bar{p}) = 1 - 0.575 = 0.425.$$

7.2. OPTIONAL TOPICS

So the multiplier is

$$\frac{0.575 \times 0.425}{(0.65 - 0.5)^2} = \frac{0.2444}{0.0225} = 10.9.$$

So (for 90% power) you multiply 21 by 10.9, giving 229 per arm.

7.1.3 Precision

Q: You wish to gather a sample to measure an expected proportion of 85% with a precision of 10%. How large should your sample be, and what will the confidence look like?

****

The required sample size is 80, and the confidence interval will be (75%, 95%).

7.2 Optional topics

7.2.1 Multiple testing

Q: A sample size for 90% power, 5% is 200 per arm. You decide to measure two outcomes which are similar and so lower the significance level to 2.5%. What will the new sample size be?

****

An increase of 18% will make it 236 per arm. However, if you had arrived at 200 after allowing for dropouts, there would be no harm in aiming for a rounder figure like 240 or even 250, which would be still better.

7.2.2 Unequal arms

Q: A trial with equal arms would have 60 per arm. Not sure that you will be able to recruit that many, you hope to make one arm 1.5 times as bigger than the other in the hope that the smaller arm will not need as many. How many can you save?

****

Here
$$k = \frac{60}{2} = 30.$$
$r = 1.5$, *so the larger arm has* $2.5 \times 30 = 75$. *For the smaller arm,*
$$\left(\frac{r+1}{r}\right) = \left(\frac{1.5+1}{1.5}\right) = \frac{5}{3}.$$
So the size of arm B is
$$\frac{5}{3} \times 30 = 50.$$
Thus you would save recruiting 10 in the smaller arm.

7.2.3 Compliance

Q: Suppose your expected size is 120, but you expect 20% of the recruits to not take treatment.

7.2. OPTIONAL TOPICS

How many will you need to recruit per arm?

****

Here $p = 0.2$, so its complement is 0.8. So we divide by $0.8^2 = 0.64$. So the size of each arm n is

$$\frac{120}{0.64} = 187.5.$$

Rounding up we get 188 per arm.

7.2.4 Clusters

Q: In a cluster trial the ICC is 0.04, and the size of the cluster is 30. What is the inflation factor? If 150 would have been needed per arm without clustering, how many clusters will you need?

****

Here $m = 30$ and $c = 0.02$, so the inflation factor is $1 + (30 - 1) \times 0.04 = 1 + 1.16 = 2.16$. We need to multiply 150 by 2.16, making 324. To get the number of clusters we divide the total number per arm by the size of each cluster:

$$\frac{324}{30} = 10.8.$$

Rounding up, you will need 11 clusters per arm.

7.2.5 Rule of 3 for rare events: confidence interval

Q: If you have 200 observations with not a single event, what will be the upper limit for the confidence interval for the proportion of rare events?

****

Here the upper limit is

$$\frac{3}{200} = 0.015.$$

So the confidence interval is (0, 0.015).

7.2.6 Rule of 3 for rare events: sample size

Q: Suppose you wanted the upper limit of the confidence interval for a rare event to be no more than 2%. How many observations will you need to have without a single event?

****

Here we have
$$\frac{3}{n} = 0.02.$$

So
$$n = \frac{3}{0.02} = 150.$$

So you will need a run of 150 observations with no events to obtain a confidence interval of (0%, 2%).

7.2. OPTIONAL TOPICS

7.2.7 Diagnostic Tests

Q: Suppose you want the lower limit of the confidence interval for the specificity of a diagnostic test to be at least to be 99.5%. How many people with a gold standard diagnosis of not having the illness will you need to test with no (false) positive test results to be sure?

****

You will need the upper confidence limit for the proportion of false positives to be 0.5%. By the Rule of 3 you need

$$\frac{3}{0.005} = 600.$$

You will need a straight run of 600 people without the condition, none of whom the test gives a false positive result for.

7.2.8 Rule of 10 for statistical modelling: sample size

Q: You wish to look at risk factors related to a condition, and you can recruit 150 people with the condition and match them with 150 who do not have it. But in advising a sponsor about prospects, you may wish to offer more conservative advice than the usual "Rule of 10". How many possible risk factors might you give the sponsor hope to find evidence for?

****

The rule tells us that you can hope to find evidence for perhaps 15 risk factors. However if you aim at something more conservative you might advise the sponsor that they shouldn't expect to find good evidence for more than about 10.

7.2.9 Before-after correlation

Q: In a before-after study, the correlation is 0.6. How much will the sample size be reduced by?

****

Here $r = 0.6$, so $r^2 = 0.36$. $1 - 0.36 = 0.64$, or 64%, which means a 36% reduction.

7.2.10 Incidence rates

Q: Suppose you want to compare two arms where the control has an incidence of 100 cases per 1000 person-years and you expect that the control has an incidence of 75 cases per 1000 person-years, but you want your investigation to pick up the difference with 90% power. You have five years to complete the study. How many people will you need to recruit in each arm to the nearest 100, assuming a dropout rate of 15%?

****

100 cases per 1000 person-years is 1 case per 10

7.2. OPTIONAL TOPICS

person-years, so your unit is 10 person-years. 75 cases per 1000 person-years is the same as 0.75 cases per 10 person-years. From the table, you will need 295 units per arm, that is 2950 person-years. You will need to recruit 590 people in each arm, apart from dropout, which are followed for five years. To allow for dropout you divide 590 by (1-0.15)=0.85, giving 694.1, or 700 per arm to the nearest 100.

7.2.11 Non-inferiority trials: Continuous Outcomes

Q: A non-inferiority trial for a continuous outcome has a tolerance of 5 units and the SD is 6.5 units. How many people will you need per arm if we aim for 90% power?

****

For 90% power the basic figure is 21. The ratio of the SD to the tolerance is 1.3, whose square is 1.69. We will need 1.69×21 = 35.49, i.e. 36 per group rounding up. In this case rounding means increasing the raw figure by more than 0.5, and so we don't need to increase it again by 1 (but there's no harm in aiming for a higher rounder figure like 40, or even 50 if we anticipate a number of dropouts.

7.2.12 Non-inferiority trials: Proportions

Q: A non-inferiority trial has a control proportion of 70% and a tolerance of 10%. For 80% power how many people will you need to recruit per arm?

****

From the table you will need 289 per arm.

7.2.13 Factorial trials

Q: A factorial term has an interaction term of 2 and the SD of all individual outcomes is 5. To detect the interaction with 80% power. how large should each arm be?

****

The ratio of the SD to I is 2.5. So you multiply the square of 2.5, which is 6.25, by 32 (for 90% power), giving 200 per arm.

Afterword

If you have worked through the previous material and tried the revision exercises as well, you should be in a good position to answer the question 'How big should my sample be?' in the main types of Medical Research studies. It is important to note, however, that for more complex studies, or measurements with an unusual distribution, the help given by this book might not be sufficient. It might be necessary to use a computer, and find the required sample size by simulation. In such cases it may be necessary to get help from a professional Statistician.

For non-statisticians who would like to learn more about the subject, I have suggested Rowntree (2018) for introductory reading. If, having finished Rowntree, you would like to try something more substantial, I would recommend Daly, Hand, Jones, Lunn, and McConway (1995). This book was originally written as the main material of an Open University course, and it is still very useful. But it assumes that you have the use of a computer. Some statistical packages can be expensive, but there are free ones available. **PSPP** in my view can be used as an accompaniment to Daly, Hand, Jones, Lunn, and McConway (1995), but its scope is naturally limited, compared to the commercial package **SPSS**. **R** is very respectable, even at research level, but has a steep learning curve, and is really for the determined student. If you want to learn it with a view to Medical applications, I would recommend Dalgaard (2008). **STATA** is expensive, but very versatile if you can get access to it.

Good luck with your researches, and remember that it is the *question* that matters. Statistics are only a means to the end of solving a scientific problem!

Technical Appendix

This part of the book is intended only for reference, and so doesn't aim at teaching. It contains some of the technical details of methods used in sample size calculation. It is in no way a comprehensive account, and interested readers may need to refer to specialist books or journals, typically found in university libraries.

1 Transformations of proportions

It is often mathematically convenient to transform proportions to derive alternative formulae for the "advantage" of one treatment over the other which we will call θ. We will use C and E to refer respectively to the Control and Experimental arms of a trial.

1. If a proportion p is left untransformed, this leads to the "advantage" being expressed as a straight difference, $\theta = p_E - p_C$.

2. inverse sine: $\arcsin(\sqrt{p})$, which leads to the "advantage" being expressed as a difference of transformed proportions,

$$\theta = \arcsin(\sqrt{p_E}) - \arcsin(\sqrt{p_C}).$$

3. log-odds[1]:
$$\ln\left(\frac{p}{1-p}\right),$$
which leads to the "advantage" being expressed as a log-odds ratio,

$$\theta = \ln\left(\frac{p_E(1-p_C)}{(1-p_E)p_C}\right).$$

2 Fisher Information and sample size

A key number in calculating sample sizes is the fraction V:
$$V = \left(\frac{U_{\frac{\alpha}{2}} + U_\beta}{\theta}\right)^2.$$

In the numerator, the Us are *upper* quantiles of the N(0,1) distribution. Thus $U_{\frac{\alpha}{2}}$ is the *upper* $100\frac{\alpha}{2}\%$ point of the Standard Normal distribution. This is the $(1 - \frac{\alpha}{2})$ Standard Normal quantile. The denominator θ is the "advantage" of the experimental treatment.

---
[1] We don't use the log-odds transformation in the main chapters, but it is included here for reference.

In Statistical terminology, V is the "Fisher information" related to a particular type of "advantage".

The sample size for each arm n then depends on the type of advantage we choose to use. Note that V is liable to be different in each case, as it depends on the type of "advantage" used.

1. Straight difference (for continuous variables):

$$n = 2\sigma^2 V,$$

where σ is the SD (derived from preliminary studies). The square of the SD is the *variance*. The "advantage" θ in this case is the difference in the means of the outcome measure across the arms.

For proportions, for values not in the tables, the approximate method taught here is based on the formulae in Altman (1991), which uses a straight difference "advantage", with an approximation being used for the overall variance of the proportions, namely $\bar{p}(1 - \bar{p})$.

2. Inverse sine transform (for proportions):

$$n = \frac{1}{2}V.$$

The inverse sine transformation is used in Matthews (2006). It was also the basis of the method we used for calculating the sample sizes for binary outcomes.

3. Log-odds transform (for proportions): we first

calculate the average proportion across the arms

$$\bar{p} = \frac{1}{2}(p_E + p_C), \text{ and then}$$

$$n = \left(\frac{2V}{\bar{p}(1-\bar{p})}\right).$$

3 Correcting for multiple testing

The crucial number here is the numerator of V, namely $(U_{\frac{\alpha}{2}} + U_\beta)^2$. For significance level 5%, power 90%, $\alpha = 0.05$ and $\beta = 0.1$. $U_{\frac{\alpha}{2}} = 1.96$ which is the upper 2.5% point (or the 0.975 Standard Normal quantile), and $U_\beta = 1.28$, which is the upper 10% point (or the 0.9 Standard Normal quantile). The critical number is therefore $(1.96 + 1.28)^2 = 10.5$.

For significance level 2.5% and the same power it is $(2.24 + 1.28)^2 = 12.4$, giving the correction factor 1.18, and hence an increase of 18%. The figure for 80% power is obtained in a similar manner.

4 Confidence intervals for proportions

A common method of finding a confidence interval for a proportion uses a Normal approximation, based on the Central Limit Theorem. An improved method by Edwin Wilson leads to asymmetric confidence intervals that are more suitable for proportions very different from 0.5. This method was used for creating the tables in this book.

5 Incidence rates

The method used for the sample size is formula (1) of Hayes and Bennett (1999).

Bibliography

Altman, D. G. (1991). *Practical Statistics for Medical Research*. Chapman and Hall.

Dalgaard, P. (2008). *Introductory Statistics with R* (Second ed.). Springer.

Daly, F., D. J. Hand, M. C. Jones, A. D. Lunn, and K. J. McConway (1995). *Elements of Statistics*. Addison-Wesley.

Eldridge, S. and S. Kerry (2012). *A Practical Guide to Cluster Randomised Trials in Health Services Research*. Wiley.

Hayes, R. and S. Bennett (1999). Sample size calculation for cluster randomized trials. *International Journal of Epidemiology 28*, 319–326.

Julious, S. A. (2023). *Sample Sizes for Clinical Trials* (Second ed.). Chapman and Hall/CRC.

Matthews, J. N. S. (2006). *Introduction to Randomized Clinical Trials* (Second ed.). CRC.

Rowntree, D. (2018). *Statistics without Tears* (Second ed.). Penguin.

Storer, B. E. (1989, September). Design and Analysis of Phase I Clinical Trials. *Biometrics 45*, 925–937.

Totton, N., J. Lin, S. Julious, M. Chowdhury, and A. Brand (2023). A review of sample sizes for UK pilot and feasibility studies on the ISRCTN registry from 2013 to 2020. *Pilot and Feasibility Studies 9*, 188.

van Belle, G. (2008). *Statistical Rules of Thumb* (Second ed.). Wiley.

TABLE Of CONTENTS

Introduction

1. Owning and renting out properties (benefits of rental income, equity building through property ownership)
2. Buying and selling properties (property flipping strategies, profit maximization)
3. Real estate development (creating value through property development)
4. Active participation in the real estate market (understanding market trends, regulatory considerations, diversifying real estate investment portfolio)
5. Investing in Real Estate Investment Trusts (REITs)

Conclusion

Introduction

Building wealth through real estate is a popular and proven system that provides people with the chance to make a constant flow of income and increase their net worth. Real estate investing offers different avenues for wealth accumulation, from possessing rental property to engaging in property and buying and selling properties for profit. This introduction will dive into the key components of building wealth through real estate and shed light on how individuals can leverage these to achieve financial success. One of the essential ways individuals build wealth through real estate is by owing and leasing properties. By acquiring Properties and renting them to tenants, individuals can generate a regular rental income, which serves as a source of passive income. This rental pay can assist with covering mortgage payments, property maintenance expenses and even provide additional income for investors. As property values appreciate over time, investors likewise benefit from equity buildings with their properties potentially increasing in value and providing a higher return on investment in the long run. Notwithstanding rental income there are ample opportunities to benefit from real estate through strategic buying and selling. Investors can distinguish undervalued properties or those with potential for development, buy them at a lower cost, and sell them at a profit after making necessary renovations or capitalizing on market trends. This methodology, known as property flipping can yield significant returns when done accurately . Real estate development presents another avenue for building wealth, By acquiring land or existing properties, investors have the opportunity to build and develop residential or commercial properties. Developing properties permits investors to create value, increase their return on investment and possibly generate huge profits when selling and renting the developed properties. Unlocking the full potential of real estate building likewise includes actively partaking in the real estate market by remaining informed about market trends, studying local regulations and analyzing investment opportunities. Diversifying a real estate investment considering various sorts of properties, for example, private , commercial or industrial can likewise contribute to wealth accumulation and provide support against market fluctuations. Furthermore, real estate investment trusts (REITs) offer people the opportunity to invest in an expanded real estate portfolio without the requirement for direct property ownership. By putting resources into public-related REITs individuals can profit from real estate income generated through an assortment of property types and locations, empowering them to access the potential for wealth accumulation in the real estate sector.

Real estate provides various avenues for building financial stability, whether through rental income, property flipping or investing in REITs.

CHAPTER ONE

Real estate investment is a popular avenue for wealth-building and financial success. One of the key strategies within real estate investment is owning and renting out properties. This involves purchasing residential or commercial properties with the intention of generating income through rental payments from tenants.

Owning and renting out properties can be a lucrative investment strategy that provides a steady stream of passive income and potential for long-term appreciation. However, it also requires careful consideration, financial planning, and active management to be successful.

When considering owning and renting out properties as a real estate investment, it's important to consider factors such as location, property type, market conditions, rental demand, and potential return on investment. These factors can determine the success and profitability of a property investment.

Additionally, owning and renting out properties also comes with operational responsibilities such as property maintenance, tenant management, lease agreements, and legal compliance. As a property owner, it's important to ensure that the property is well-maintained, and tenants' needs are met to maximize rental income and maintain property value.

From a financial perspective, owning and renting out properties can provide investors with a reliable income stream, tax advantages, and potential appreciation in property value over time. However, it's crucial to carefully assess the costs associated with property ownership and rental management, as well as potential risks such as vacancy rates, property damage, and changes in market conditions.

Owning and renting out properties in real estate investment can be a rewarding and profitable venture for those who are willing to take on the responsibilities of property ownership and management. With careful planning and strategic decision-making, investors can enjoy the benefits of passive income, capital appreciation, and long-term wealth accumulation through real estate rental properties.

Benefits of Rental Income

What is ROI?

ROI, which stands for return on investment, is the probability of gaining a profit from the total money invested. When investing in a rental property, the amount of money coming in and going out (i.e. the cash flow) may provide a net gain or loss. The goal of rental property investing is to generate a positive cash flow, so the amount of money earned on the property is greater than the expenses going into managing the property.

Cost of investment

The amount of money spent on the rental property is considered the total cost of investment. Here are some of the expenses you'll likely see as a rental property owner:

Purchase price: The amount paid by the investor for the rental property. The purchase price can be paid for in cash or be financed through a mortgage lender.

Down payment: A percentage of the purchase price that is paid upfront by the investor. A down payment between 20% and 30% is generally required for a rental property that will be rented out from day one.

Mortgage interest: The annual cost to borrow money from a lender, expressed as a percentage rate.

Property tax: A tax expense paid on owned property. Property tax, which is usually based on the value of the property and land, may fluctuate.

Insurance: Homeowners insurance protects the property owner's liability and insures the residence against damages and losses. The average annual premium on home insurance usually costs less than 1% of the purchase price. With rental property, there may be additional insurance coverage needed.

Operating expenses Typically, the cost to operate a rental property is around 35% to 85% of the rental income or 1% of the property value per year. Operating expenses may include repair costs, maintenance costs, property management fees, HOA fees, advertising costs, utility costs or vacancy costs.

Gains on investment

The amount of money earned from the rental property is considered the total investment gain or profit. Here are the typical gains that may come out of a rental property investment:

Rent: A tenant's regular monthly payment to a landlord for the use of the property or land. Rent is generally the primary source of income on a rental property.

Appreciation: The increase in value of a property over time, expressed as an annual percentage rate. As a home rises in value, the investor can earn profit from the appreciation. The national appreciation value averages at around 3.5% to 3.8% per year.

Additional rental income: Any additional money earned from the tenant like income from utilities, laundry, storage or parking fees.

How to calculate ROI on rental property

First, calculate the return on investment by subtracting the total gains from the cost. Then, divide the total return by the cost of investment to calculate the rental property ROI.

(Cost of Investment- Gains on Investment)/Cost of Investment = ROI

To convert the rental ROI to a percentage multiply it by 100.

ROI * 100 = ROI percentage

For example, if you invest $50,000 in a rental property and get a profit of $70,000, the ROI would be 0.4 or 40%.

($70,000 – $50,000) / $50,000 = 0.4   0.4 * 100 = 40%

Rental income can offer a large number of benefits for people, investors, and even organizations. Here is a broad exploration of some of these benefits:

Consistent Income

One of the clearest advantages of rental income is the steady cash flow it can provide. With reliable tenants, property owners can depend on a regular stream of income, which can assist with covering mortgage payments, and property upkeep expenses, and even generate passive income.

Appreciation:

Real Estate properties by and large will generally increase in value over the long run, which can expand the worth of the rental property. This appreciation can prompt significant profits from investment, particularly if the property is situated in a popular region or encounters a huge turn of events and infrastructure improvements.

Tax Benefits:

Rental income frequently accompanies different tax advantages. Property owners can deduct expenses, for example, mortgage interest, property taxes, insurance, maintenance, and devaluation. Moreover, there are tax benefits related to rental property ownership, such as the ability to defer capital gain taxes through 1031 exchanges and the deduction of rental losses against different sources of income for qualified investors.

Portfolio Diversification

Investing resources into rental properties permits individuals to diversify their investment portfolio. Real Estate typically acts differently in contrast to stocks, bonds, and other traditional investments, providing support against market unpredictability and economic downturns.

Inflation Hedge:

Rental income can act as a hedge against inflation. As the cost of living increases, rental prices will rise too, allowing property owners to change their rental rates accordingly and maintain the purchasing power of their income.

Asset Appreciation:

Beyond cash flow, rental properties can appreciate over time, giving owners capital appreciation. This appreciation can result from different factors, such as market demand, neighborhood developments, renovations, and enhancements to the actual property.

Control Over Investment:

Dissimilar to other investment vehicles like stocks or mutual funds, owning rental property gives investors more control over their investment. Property owners can make decisions regarding property management, tenant selection, rental pricing, and property improvements, permitting them to improve their profits and mitigate risks.

Leverage:

Real Estate investors can use their investment by supporting the acquisition of rental properties through mortgages. By using borrowed capital, investors can multiply their profits and increase their purchasing power, possibly accelerating wealth accumulation.

Retirement Income:

Rental income can act as a dependable source of retirement income. By owning rental properties or having them mostly paid off by the time of retirement, individuals can enjoy a constant flow of income to enhance other retirement savings and social security benefits.

Legacy Building:

Rental properties can be passed down to future generations, serving as a legacy for heirs. Real estate assets can provide long-term financial security for beneficiaries and continue to generate income for years to come. Rental income offers a range of benefits, including consistent income, appreciation potential, tax benefits, diversification, inflation security, and control over investments, making it an alluring option for investors seeking steady income and long-term wealth accumulation.

Equity Building through Property Ownership

Homeownership comes with major perks. It allows you to establish your unique living environment and an increased level of financial stability. It additionally offers you the ability to build equity in your home. Equity is the contrast between the amount of money that you owe the mortgage lender and how much cash your house is worth. Over time, you will make mortgage payments on the house, decreasing the loan's principal balance, thus building equity by increasing the percentage of the home you own.

How does equity function?

If you were to buy a home worth $300,000, for instance, using a $30,000 down payment, you would consequently have $30,000 of equity at closing. As you make each payment toward your mortgage, your loan balance will decrease. This develops more equity as long as the worth of your home remains the same or increments over the long run. When you pay 100% of your mortgage, you will have 100% equity. Sometimes, home prices can drop sharply, and a homeowner might owe the lender more than whatever the house is worth. Using our model, assuming the home's value dropped to $200,000 you still owed $240,000, the loan would be considered "underwater," or you would have "negative equity."

How would you build equity in your home?

There are a few unique ways of developing value in your home, including:

- Increasing the down payment you put on your home at the time of purchase.
. Increasing your mortgage payment amount or making additional payments.
- Renegotiation and shortening the term of your loan.
- Investing in home improvement and remodeling projects to Increase the home's value.

The most ideal way to the equity of a home

You can take advantage of the equity of a home you have built as a minimal expense and convenient way to borrow money and take advantage of a great interest rate.

Depending on a person's credit score and financial history, that implies their home equity is at 20% or more before the bank/lender permits them to borrow against the value of their home. Lenders will typically allow you to borrow up to 80% of the total value of your home. Most home equity loan terms will range between five and 20 years. But borrows can take 30 years to pay a home equity loan. Since a lot of a borrower's monthly loan payment goes straightforwardly to interest payments at the beginning of the loan term. It can take five to seven years before a mortgage holder can reach the 20% equity limit. There are a few reasons why you would use your home equity to borrow money, for example, to cover business expenses. Numerous entrepreneurs will take advantage of home equity and use the cash to assist with developing their businesses. The move is especially beneficial while keeping away from higher financing costs associated with a small business loan.

Finance Emergency Expenses

Emergencies occur. Most financial advisors propose having a just-in-case account covering six months of your living expenses. But, that is hard for most people to do. A home equity loan might be your best decision when confronted with a crisis and no way to get the funds you need.

Consolidate your Debt

Home equity loans can be great tools for merging high-interest debts at lower interest rates. You can utilize this strategy to assist you with paying off personal debts like credit cards and car loans.

Pay for College

Assuming the moneylender approves, you can use your home equity to cover college expenses. Even though student loans are usually your best bet for paying college expenses, home equity loans can sometimes offer better low-interest options.

Finance Home Upgrades

Home equity loans are most commonly used for home improvement projects because, in addition to making your home more decent, comfortable, and alluring, the upgrades that you make might raise the house's value, thus building more equity. It can truly be a win-win. There is no doubt that most Americans who can buy a home do so to put a roof over their heads. In any case, through equity, homeownership genuinely becomes an investment.

A home equity loan serves as a valuable tool for the responsible homeowner who needs to cash. Low-interest rates and tax deduction opportunities make a home equity loan an excellent choice for any homeowner. They simply need to ensure they have a steady income that can repay the loan.

property ownership serves as a strong vehicle for building equity and achieving long-term financial stability. Property ownership, first and foremost, allows individuals to build equity through the gradual repayment of mortgage loans. Each mortgage payment made contributes to lessening the outstanding loan balance, thereby increasing the homeowner's equity stake in the property. Over time, as the home loan is settled, the equity of the property grows, providing homeowners with valuable assets that can be leveraged for future investment or financial needs.

Additionally, property appreciation plays a significant role in equity building. Real estate properties have historically appreciated over the long term, driven by factors, such as market demand, inflation, and neighborhood development. As property values increase, homeowners see a corresponding increase in their equity position, allowing them to build wealth passively without extra effort. Moreover, strategic property upgrades and renovation can additionally improve equity growth. By investing in upgrades that increment the property's value, homeowners can speed up equity building and maximize their returns on the investment. These improvements add to property appreciation as well as improve the overall desirability and marketability of the property, potentially attracting higher rental income or resale values. Furthermore, home ownership offers tax advantages that can boost equity-building efforts. Deductions for mortgage interest, property taxes, and home improvement can assist homeowners with reducing their tax liabilities, allowing them to allocate more resources towards mortgage payments or equity-building investments. Also, certain tax-deferred exchanges, like the 1031 exchange, provide opportunities for homeowners to reinvest proceeds from property sales into higher-value properties without immediate tax consequences.

Equity Vs. Debt Investments for Real Estate

There are two primary ways of investing in real estate: through equity or debt. Equity investments commonly include purchasing a piece of property and becoming a part-owner, while debt investments involve lending cash to borrowers who buy a property with the expectation of earning interest on that loan. Both have their unique pros and cons. The primary contrast in real estate investment strategy boils down to where you sit in the capital stack. The capital stack is the order in which debt and equity are layered in a real estate deal. The most important thing to remember about the capital stack is that status matters — in case of a default, lenders who have rank will be first in line to get paid back. This is why you normally see a correlation between the level of risk you take on and the reward.

Equity Investments

With equity investments, you are purchasing a piece of the property and becoming a part owner. This type of investment is typically riskier because you own the property and hold on to the liability of ownership. On the off chance that the property appreciates, you will probably see a bigger profit from your investment. Equity investments ordinarily have a more extended holding period than some debt instruments, so you ought to expect to see potentially larger returns for longer periods of illiquidity.

Debt Investment

Another way to invest in a commercial real estate capital stack is to participate on the debt side. With debt investment, generally, you are lending money to a borrower with the expectation of being paid your principal plus interest. This type of investment is typically safer than equity since you are not directly owning the property, and in most cases will have the underlying asset as collateral. Nonetheless, if the borrower defaults on their loan, you could shoulder the burden of having to work out the rest of the deal to recover your principal. Debt improvement may have a shorter holding period than equity, depending on the type of debt. You should expect to see more consistent repayment though so you can anticipate some form of return soon.

Diversifying Your Investment Portfolio

Regardless of which type of investment you choose, diversifying your investment portfolio is important. This implies investing in different types of assets to mitigate risk. For instance, if you are only investing in equity, you could be putting all your eggs in one basket. Equity investments fluctuate with their respective markets while debt investments tend to remain all the more balanced. In any case, if you expand and choose to invest in both equity and debt, you'll help balance out the risk and possibly increase your probability of reaching the investment objective.

CHAPTER TWO

Buying and Selling Properties

Real estate investing is the purchase of real estate. To fully comprehend this definition, we must first define real estate. Real estate is basically any piece of land and property attached to that land. Anything natural or man-made that is a part of this land, including trees, buildings, or fences, is viewed as real estate. You could hear individuals use the words land, real estate, and real property interchangeably. However, there are slight differences between each term. The land is any natural surface and airspace — whatever you could attribute to being a part of Mother Earth. Real estate is this land plus any permanent man-made addition, like a home. Finally, real property is the set of incentives and benefits from owning real estate. Consequently, investing in real estate into land is the act of purchasing a piece of land plus any man-made additions made to that land. There are several categories of real estate investing, and the most well known ones are residential, commercial, and industrial real estate investing. Investing in real estate can appear to be costly at first, however it is one of the most demonstrated ways of creating financial stability.

Property Flipping Strategies Property flipping is a popular investment strategy where investors buy a property with the intention of reselling it quickly for a profit. It requires cautious planning and execution. Here's an extensive guide to follow:

Market Research: Begin by educating yourself about the real estate market. Understand the different types of properties, market trends, financing options, and investment strategies. Research various areas and regions to identify areas with growth potential, rental demand, or resale value appreciation.

Define Your Investment Goals: Determine your investment objectives, whether it's long-term wealth accumulation, automated income through rental properties, or short-term flipping for profit. Set financial goals, including target returns on investment, cash flow requirement, and risk tolerance.

Financial Planning: Evaluate your financial situation and decide your budget for investment. Explore financial options like mortgages, loans, or partnerships. Calculate expected profits on investment, factoring in expenses like property taxes, insurance, maintenance and vacancy rates.

Property Search and Due Diligence: Start looking for properties that align with your investment criteria. Consider factors, such as, location, property type, condition, and potential for appreciation. Conduct thorough due diligence, including property inspections, title searches, zoning regulations, and potential liabilities. Assess the property's income potential by analyzing by rental income, vacancy rates, and operating expenses.

Negotiation and Acquisition

Make an offer based on your research and analysis. Negotiate terms like cost, closing date, possibilities, and financing arrangements. Work with realtors, attorneys, or advisors to facilitate the purchase and process and ensure legal compliance. Secure financing and finalize the purchase agreement, ensuring all important documentation is in order.

Property Management (for Rental properties)

If investing in rental properties, develop a management plan for tenant screening, lease agreements, rent collection, maintenance, and repairs. Consider hiring a property management company to handle day-to-day operations if you prefer a hands-off approach.

Investment Exit Strategy

Decide your exit strategy, whether it's selling the property for profit, refinancing to leverage equity, or holding for long-term appreciation. Monitor market conditions and property performance regularly to assess the best time to sell or refinance.

Marketing and Sales (for Selling)

If selling a property, prepare it for sale by making necessary repairs, organizing, and upgrading curb appeal. Develop a marketing strategy to attract potential buyers, utilizing online listings, open houses, signage, and professional photography. Consider hiring a realtor to facilitate the sales process, negotiate offers, and handle paperwork.

Closing the Deal

Review and negotiate offers from potential buyers, considering factors like price, contingencies, and closing timelines. Work with a real estate attorney or closing agent to finalize the transaction, ensuring all legal requirements are met. Transfer ownership, exchange funds, and complete all necessary documentation to close the deal.

Learn and Adapt

Reflect on each investment experience to identify lessons learned and areas for improvement. Stay informed about market trends, regulatory changes, and investment strategies to adjust your approach accordingly.

How and When to Maximize Profit

Boosting profit through trading involves several key strategies aimed at acquiring properties at a great cost selling them at a favorable price and selling them at a higher value. Here is a detailed outline of these strategies:

Purchase Below Market Value Search for properties priced below their market worth due to distress, foreclosure, or motivated sellers. Negotiate effectively to secure the best possible purchase price. Consider factors, such as property condition, location, and market demand when evaluating a potential deal.

Renovation and Value-Add

Invest in renovation and improvements that significantly increase the property's value. Focus on upgrades with high return on investment (ROI) such as kitchen and bathroom remodels, energy-efficient upgrades, and cosmetic enhancements. Prioritize projects that enhance curb appeal and overall functionality.

Target Undervalued Properties Identify properties with undiscovered potential or overlooked features that can be leveraged to increase their worth. This could include properties in up-and-coming neighborhoods, homes with unique architectural features, or properties with development potential (e.g., partitioning land).

Timing the Market

Monitor market trends and timing to capitalize on favorable conditions. Buy properties during periods of low demand or economic downturns when prices are depressed. Aim to sell during peak seasons or when market conditions favor sellers to maximize selling costs.

Strategic Financing

Secure financing with ideal terms to limit borrowing costs and augment returns. Explore options like traditional mortgages, private loans, or hard money lenders, depending on the project's requirements and your financial situation. Consider leveraging other people's money (OPM) to increase purchasing power and ROI.

Minimize Holding Costs

Limit holding costs by completing renovations rapidly and efficiently. Avoid over-improving the property beyond what is necessary to attract

buyers. Set realistic timelines for renovation projects and effectively oversee contractors to stay on schedule. Additionally, explore choices to decrease carrying costs such as short-term financing or leasing the property during the selling process.

Effective Marketing and Sales Strategies

Develop a comprehensive marketing plan to attract potential buyers and create competition. Use professional photography, staging, virtual tours, and online postings to showcase the property's features. Implement targeted advertising campaigns and use social media and networking channels to reach a wider audience.

Price Strategically

Set the selling price based on market comparables, property condition, and buyer demand. Avoid overpricing, which can dissuade buyers or underpricing. Consider pricing competitively to generate various offers and create a sense of urgency among buyers.

Negotiation Skills

Improve your negotiation skills to maximize profit during both the buying and selling phases. Negotiate aggressively when buying properties to secure favorable terms and pricing. During the selling process, haggle with buyers to achieve the highest possible selling price while ensuring a smooth exchange.

Continuous Learning and Adaptation

Remain informed about market trends, industry best practices, and evolving strategies for trading properties. Consistently assess your performance, learn from successes and failures, and adjust your strategies accordingly to stay competitive and maximize profitability.

Timing

The timing for maximizing real estate profits can vary depending on different factors like location, economic situations, and property type. However, there are generally a few trends to consider:

Spring: In many regions, the spring season is considered one of the best times to sell real estate. Warmer weather and longer sunshine hours tend to attract more buyers, leading to increased competition and possibly higher selling prices. Additionally, families often prefer to move during the spring and summer months to avoid disrupting the school year.

Summer: The summer months can likewise be ideal for real estate deals, especially in areas with a strong vacation or second-home market. Buyers may be more active during this time, taking advantage of their time off to search for properties. Outdoor spaces and amenities tend to be more appealing during the summer, potentially driving up property values.

Early Fall: The early fall season can be another good time for real estate deals, as buyers who missed out on summer deals may still be actively searching. Also, families planning to move before the start of the new school year may be eager to finalize purchases during this time.

Market Dynamics

While these seasons generally see increased buyer activity, it's essential to consider local market dynamics. In some regions, for example, areas with mild climate or strong tourism, the real estate market may remain active year-round. On the other hand, in colder climates, the market might dial back during the winter months.

Seller's Market Vs. Buyer's Market The condition of the market can likewise influence the timing for maximizing profits. In a seller's market, where demand exceeds supply, sellers may have more flexibility in choosing when to list their properties and may be able to command higher prices regardless of the season. In contrast, in a buyer's market, where inventory is high and demand is low, sellers may need to be more strategic about timing their listings to maximize profit. Eventually, while certain seasons might offer better conditions for real estate deals, the key is to carefully survey local market trends, consider the specific attributes of the property being sold, and decisively time the listing to capitalize on peak buyer demand and market dynamics. Moreover, factors such as interest rates, economic conditions, and regulatory changes can also influence the timing for boosting real estate profits.

CHAPTER THREE

Real Estate Development

There are several types of real estate investors should be familiar with. Each of these types will come with unique advantages and disadvantages that investors should evaluate. Let's look at each option available:

1. Residential Real Estate

2. Commercial Real Estate

3. Crude Land and New Construction

4. Real Estate Investment Trusts (REITs)

5. Crowdfunding Platforms

1. Residential Real Estate. There are various rental property types in residential real estate, though the most common is believed to be single-family homes. Other residential properties include duplexes, multifamily properties, and vacation homes. Residential real estate is ideal for some investors because it can be easy to turn profits consistently. There are numerous residential real estate investing strategies to deploy and different levels of competition across markets — what might be

appropriate for one investor may not be best for the next. For this reason, choosing the right exit strategy and market is key when it comes to residential real estate. The most common exit strategies used in residential real estate include wholesaling, rehabbing, and purchasing and holding properties, which can be used to generate rental income. Investors ought to be mindful to consider which strategies would work best in their market area by conducting a thorough market analysis. When managed correctly, a residential real estate investment can yield good profits. This is because, in addition to earning steady cash flow, residential real estate benefits from several tax breaks.

2. Commercial Real Estate. The best commercial properties to invest in include industrial, office, retail, accommodation, and multifamily projects. For investors with a strong focus on improving their local communities, commercial real estate investing can support that focus. One reason commercial properties are considered one of the best types of real estate investments is the potential for higher cash flow. Investors who opt for commercial properties may find they represent higher income potential, longer leases, and lower vacancy than other forms of real estate. Industrial real estate includes warehouses, storage units, car washes, and other special-purpose properties that produce revenue from clients who visit the facility. Industrial real estate investments frequently include major fee

and service revenue streams, such as coin-operated vacuum cleaners at a car wash, which can help the owner maximize their return on investment. Investors may also enjoy less competition in commercial real estate because purchasing these properties can be a larger undertaking than working with residential homes. To learn more about getting started, be sure to read this book.

3. Crude Land Investing and New Construction

Crude land investing and new construction represent two types of real estate investment that can diversify an investor's portfolio. Crude land refers to any vacant land available for purchase and is most attractive in markets with high projected growth. New construction isn't very different; however, properties have already been built on the land. Investing in new construction is also popular in rapidly growing markets. While numerous financial backers may be unfamiliar with crude land and new construction investing, these investment types can represent attractive profits for investors. appealing benefits for financial backers. Whether you are keen on developing a property from start to finish or profiting from a long-term purchase and hold, crude land and new construction provide a good opportunity for real estate investors. Investors should be prepared to complete extensive market research to maximize profits when investing in crude land and new construction. This will ensure you choose a desirable area and prevent the investment from being hampered by market factors.

4. Real Estate Investment Trusts(REITs)

Real estate investment trusts or REITs are companies that own different commercial real estate types, such as hotels, shops, offices, shopping malls, or restaurants. You can invest in shares of these real estate companies on the stock exchange. when you invest in a REIT, you invest in the properties these companies own without the added risk of owning the property yourself. It is a requirement for REITs to return 90% of their taxable income to shareholders every year. This allows investors to receive dividends while diversifying their portfolios Publicly traded REITs also offer flexible liquidity in contrast to other types of real estate investment. You can sell your shares of the company on the stock exchange when you need emergency funds.

5. Crowdfunding Platforms

Crowdfunding platforms offer investors access to several assets that offer high returns and are traditionally reserved for the wealthy. While this offers the ease of finding assets to investors, this type of real estate also introduces a high amount of risk. Crowdfunding platforms are typically limited to accredited investors or those with a high net worth. Some sites offer access to non-accredited investors as well. The main types of real estate investment from crowdfunding platforms are non-traded REITs or REITs that are not on the stock exchange. In terms of non-traded REITs, your funds may be invested for several years with no possibility of pulling your money out when you need it.

What Is the Best Type of Real Estate Investment?

The best type of real estate investment will depend on your conditions, goals, market area, and preferred investing strategy. While many investors need a more clear response, determining the best type of investment property is a subjective process. Choosing the right property type comes down to weighing each option's pros and cons, though there are a few key factors investors should keep in mind as they seek the best choice. When choosing the best type of investment property, the importance of location cannot be understated. Investors operating in "up-and-coming" markets may find success with vacant land or new construction, while investors working in more "mature" markets may be interested in residential properties. Aside from location, investors should be aware of their preferences when it comes to investing. Assess your preferred level of involvement, risk tolerance, and profitability as you decide which property type to invest in. Investors wishing to take on a more passive role may opt to buy and hold commercial or residential properties and employ a property manager. Those hoping to take on a more active role, on the other hand, may find developing vacant land or rehabbing residential homes to be more fulfilling. As you choose the best type of investment property for you, it is important to keep in mind that many investors find success investing in various property types. It is not uncommon for investors to familiarize themselves with residential real estate before moving on to commercial properties. That being said, there is no reason investors cannot achieve success investing in multiple property types.

Active Vs. Passive Investing

An important distinction to make

when choosing an investment strategy is between active and passive investments. Active strategies, as the name implies, require a more hands-on management approach. For instance, rehabbing a house is considered an active investment strategy. You will be in charge of coordinating renovations, overseeing contractors, and ultimately ensuring the property sells. Active strategies demand more time and effort, though they are related with large profit margins. On the other hand, passive real estate investing is great for investors who want to take a less elaborate approach. Examples of passive real estate investing include REITs, buy and holds, or rental property ownership. With these strategies, you can enjoy passive income over time while allowing your investments to be managed by someone else (such as a property management company). The main thing to remember is that you can lose out on some of your returns by hiring someone else to manage the investment. Generally, the right investment approach will depend on your schedule, skill level, and finances.

Direct Vs. Indirect Investing

Another consideration to make when selecting a real estate investing strategy is direct vs. indirect. Similar to active vs. passive investing, direct vs. indirect refers to the level of involvement required. Direct investments involve actually purchasing or managing properties, while indirect strategies are less hands on. For instance, REIT investing or crowdfunded properties are indirect real estate investments. Direct investments include buying or rehabbing.

Where To Find Real Estate Investment Properties

Many investors can get so caught up in identifying a property type that they don't have any idea where to begin when it comes to finding an actual property. So as you look into different property types, also be certain to learn where and how to find each one. Here are a few options investors may find useful: MLS Listings and FSBOs : MLS means Multiple Listing Service, it is an database established by real estate brokers to provide data about properties for sale. FSBO (for sale by the owner) This shows that a property is available for purchase directly from the owner rather than through a realtor or a broker. This help you to avoid paying agents commissions. Many investors find properties on the MLS or FSBO listing. There are tons of properties available that remain unnoticed because investors and homebuyers don't know where to look. Some of these properties suffer from poor or non-existent marketing, while others are overpriced when listed and therefore failed to receive any attention. This implies that those investors willing to sort through the MLS can find a variety of investment opportunities. To access MLS, investors either need to be a realtor themselves or willing to work with one. This way, investors can consistently track or be alerted to new listings in their target area. For those wondering how to make connections with realtors in their respective areas, it is a good idea to attend local networking or real estate event. Investors looking for FSBO properties in a given area and may be willing to pass that information to their investor partners. Investors can can also drive through their target areas, looking for signs to find these properties. Keep in mind, identifying properties can take time, and investors should be ready to employ multiple angles to secure their next deal.

Off-Market Properties

For investors living in oversaturated markets, off-market properties can present an opportunity to get ahead of the competition. However they are not listed on the MLS, off-market properties are not difficult to find; investors need to know how to search. With regards to searching for off-market properties, there are a few resources investors should check first. These include public records, real estate auctions, wholesalers, networking events, and contractors. Every of these sources presents a unique chance to find properties in a given area. For example, wholesalers are often aware of newly rehabbed properties available at reasonable prices. Many of these are already leased — and may even come with an existing property management company. Then there are foreclosures. Despite numerous proclamations in the news that foreclosures are vanishing, data from Realty Trac continues to show spikes in activity around the world. Years of backlogged foreclosures and increased motivation for banks to repossess could leave even more foreclosures up for grabs in the coming months. Investors searching for foreclosures should pay careful attention to newspaper listings and public records to find potential properties. Overall, off-market properties are not to find, however they might require a little extra work.

How Do You Invest In Real Estate?

Real estate investing is the purchase of real estate. To completely understand this definition, we must first define real estate. Real Estate is essentially any piece of land and property attached to that land. Anything natural or man-made that is part of this land, including trees, buildings, or fences is considered Real Estate. You could hear people use the words land, real estate, and real property conversely. In any case, there are slight differences between each term. The land is any natural surface and airspace — anything you could attribute to being part of Mother Earth. Real estate Land is this land plus any permanent man-made additions, like a home. Finally, real property is the set of incentives and benefits from owning real estate. Thus investing in real estate

is the act of purchasing a piece of land plus any man-made additions made to that land. There are several categories of real estate investing, and the most popular ones are residential, commercial, and industrial real estate. Investing in real estate can seem expensive at first, but it is one of the most proven ways to build wealth. We discuss how you can make money by investing in real estate next.

CHAPTER FOUR

Active Participation In Real Estate Market

You can be eligible as an active participant in real estate if you own 10% or more of the rental property, have significant involvement in the management of the rental property, and are not a limited partner.

With active participation in real estate, you may be eligible to deduct up to $25,000 from your rental real estate in passive losses each year from non-passive income. Passive and non-passive income in real estate are two fundamental concepts that investors should understand to optimize their investment strategies. Here's an extensive breakdown of each:

Passive Income in Real Estate:

Definition: Passive income refers to earnings derived from rental properties or real estate investments where the investor is not actively involved in day-to-day management or operations. It provides a steady stream of income without requiring significant ongoing effort.

Examples:

1. Rental Properties: Income generated from tenants paying rent on residential or commercial properties.

2. Real Estate Investment Trusts (REITs): Investors can earn passive income by investing in REITs, which are companies that own, operate, or finance income-producing real estate.

3. Real Estate Crowdfunding: Through online platforms, investors can pool funds to invest in real estate projects, earning passive income from rental income or property appreciation.

Advantages:

1. Steady Cash Flow: Rental properties can provide a consistent stream of income, which can be especially beneficial for retirement planning or financial stability.

2. Tax Benefits: Real estate investments offer various tax advantages, including depreciation deductions, mortgage interest deductions, and the ability to defer capital gains taxes through 1031 exchanges.

3. Diversification: Real estate can serve as a hedge against stock market volatility, offering diversification within an investment portfolio.

Challenges:

1. Initial Capital Requirement: Acquiring rental properties often requires a significant upfront investment, which may be prohibitive for some investors.

2. Property Management: While passive, real estate investments still require some level of management, such as

dealing with tenants, property maintenance, and potential vacancies.

3. Market Risk: Real estate values can fluctuate based on economic conditions, interest rates, and local market dynamics, impacting the profitability of investments.

Non-Passive Income in Real Estate:

Definition: Non-passive income involves actively participating in real estate activities, such as property flipping, real estate development, or real estate brokerage. It typically requires hands-on involvement and effort from the investor.

Examples:

1. Property Flipping: Buying distressed properties, renovating them, and selling them for a profit.

2. Real Estate Development: Investing in the construction or redevelopment of properties, such as residential communities, commercial buildings, or mixed-use developments.

3. Real Estate Brokerage: Earning commissions by facilitating property transactions as a licensed real estate agent or broker.

Advantages:

1. Higher Profit Potential: Non-passive real estate activities often offer higher profit margins compared to passive income strategies, particularly in property flipping or development projects.

2. Control: Investors have greater control over the outcome of their investments and can directly influence property value

through renovations, improvements, or strategic development decisions.

3. Flexibility: While it requires active involvement, non-passive real estate activities can offer flexibility in terms of project selection, timing, and execution.

Challenges:

1. Time and Effort: Non-passive real estate activities demand a significant time commitment and expertise in areas such as property valuation, construction management, and market analysis.

2. Market Volatility: Fluctuations in the real estate market, construction costs, and regulatory changes can introduce uncertainty and risk to non-passive real estate investments.

3. Capital Intensity: Many non-passive real estate activities require substantial capital investment, including financing for property acquisitions, construction costs, and carrying expenses during project development.

Both passive and non-passive income strategies offer distinct advantages and challenges in real estate investing. Passive income provides steady cash flow with minimal ongoing effort, while non-passive income offers higher profit potential but requires active involvement and expertise. Investors should carefully evaluate their financial goals, risk tolerance, and resources when deciding between these two approaches.

Understanding Market Trends

! Understanding market trends is essential for making informed decisions in various industries, including real estate, finance, retail, and technology. By analyzing market trends, businesses and investors can anticipate shifts in consumer behavior, identify emerging opportunities, and adapt their strategies to remain competitive. Here's an extensive overview of how to understand market trends effectively:

1. Data Analysis:

Quantitative Data: Utilize quantitative data such as sales figures, market shares, revenue growth rates, and demographic statistics to identify patterns and trends.

Qualitative Data: Supplement quantitative data with qualitative insights from customer feedback, industry reports, expert opinions, and market surveys to gain a comprehensive understanding of market dynamics.

2. Economic Indicators:

Macro-Economic Indicators: Monitor macro-economic indicators such as GDP growth, inflation rates, unemployment rates, interest rates, and consumer confidence levels to assess the overall health of the economy and its impact on market trends.

Industry-specific Indicators: Identify industry-specific economic indicators relevant to your sector, such as housing starts, construction spending, retail sales, or manufacturing output, to gauge industry performance and anticipate market trends.

3. Technological Innovations:

Emerging Technologies: Stay abreast of technological innovations and advancements in your industry, such as artificial intelligence, blockchain, Internet of Things (IoT), and renewable energy, as these can disrupt traditional business models and create new market opportunities.

Adoption Rates: Monitor the adoption rates of new technologies among consumers and businesses to identify trends and assess the potential impact on market dynamics.

4. Consumer Behavior:

Demographic Shifts: Understand demographic trends such as population growth, aging populations, urbanization, and changing household structures to tailor products and services to evolving consumer needs.

Psychographic Segmentation: Segment consumers based on psychographic factors such as lifestyle preferences, values, attitudes, and behaviors to target specific market segments effectively.

Consumer Preferences: Analyze consumer preferences, buying habits, and purchasing patterns through market research, social media analytics, and sales data to identify emerging trends and adapt marketing strategies accordingly.

5. Competitive Landscape:

Competitor Analysis: Conduct a thorough analysis of competitors, including their products, pricing strategies, marketing tactics, and market share, to benchmark performance and identify areas for differentiation.

SWOT Analysis: Evaluate the strengths, weaknesses, opportunities, and threats (SWOT) facing your business and its competitors to identify strategic advantages and potential risks in the market.

6. Regulatory Environment:

Legal and Regulatory Changes: Stay informed about changes in the regulatory environment, including new laws, policies, and compliance requirements that may impact your industry, market dynamics, and business operations.

Industry Standards: Adhere to industry standards, certifications, and best practices to maintain compliance, enhance credibility, and mitigate regulatory risks.

7. Global Trends: Globalization: Consider global trends and developments, such as international trade agreements, geopolitical tensions, currency fluctuations, and emerging markets, that may influence your industry and market trends.

Supply Chain Disruptions: Assess the impact of global events, natural disasters, pandemics, and supply chain disruptions on production, distribution, and market dynamics to mitigate risks and identify opportunities for resilience.

8. Environmental and Social Factors:

Sustainability: Embrace environmental sustainability and corporate social responsibility (CSR) practices to align with consumer preferences, regulatory requirements, and market trends towards eco-friendly products and ethical business practices.

Social Trends: Monitor social trends, cultural shifts, and lifestyle changes that may influence consumer behavior, product demand, and market preferences, such as health and wellness, diversity and inclusion, and ethical consumption.

Understanding market trends requires a holistic approach that integrates data analysis, economic indicators, technological innovations, consumer behavior, competitive analysis, regulatory compliance, global trends, and environmental and social factors. By continuously monitoring and analyzing market trends, businesses and investors can anticipate changes, seize opportunities, and adapt their strategies to play dynamic and competitive markets.

Regulatory Considerations for Real Estate Investment

Regulatory considerations plays a crucial role in real estate, ate management of the legal framework within which investors operate, and can significantly impact investment decisions, property development, financing, and ongoing management. Here is a broad outline of regulatory considerations of real estate investment:

1. Zoning and Land Use Regulations

Zoning Laws: Understand local zoning regulations that designate how land can be used, including residential, commercial, industrial, or mixed-use zoning districts. Land Use Restrictions: Be aware of land use restrictions, setback requirements, building height limits, and other zoning ordinances that might affect property development and usage.

2. Building Code and Permitting Building Standards: Comply with building codes and construction standards set by local building departments to ensure structural integrity, permits and compliance with health and environmental regulations.

Permitting Process: Acquire necessary approval and permits for construction, renovations, alterations, changes in land use from relevant authorities to avoid legal liabilities and fines.

3. Environmental Regulations Environmental Assessments: Conduct environmental assessments, such as Phase 1 Environmental Site Assessments (ESAs), to identify possible contamination materials, or natural liabilities associated with the property.

Environmental Remediation: Address environmental issues through remediation endeavors, cleanup activities, or compliance with environmental regulations to mitigate risks and protect public health and the environment.

4. Landlord-Tenant Laws

Lease Agreement Draft: lease arrangements that comply with landlord-tenant laws governing rental properties, including lease terms, rent increments, security deposits, eviction procedures, and tenant rights.

Fair Housing Act: Adhere to the Fair Housing Act and other anti-discrimination laws based on race, color, religion, anti-discrimination national origin, or disability in housing transactions.

5. Tax Considerations

Property Taxes: Understand property tax assessments and valuation methods, understanding can impact investment returns and methods. Tax Incentives: Take advantages of tax advantage deductions, capital gains exclusions, and tax-deferred exchanges (e.g., 1031 exchanges).

6. Financing and Mortgage Regulations

Lending Regulations: Comply with lending regulations, mortgage disclosure requirements, and consumer protection laws governing real estate financing, including Truth in Lending Act (TILA), Real Estate Settlement Act(RESPA), and Dodd-Frank Act.

Loan Terms: Understand loan terms, interest rates, amortization schedules, prepayment penalties, and loan-to-value ratios when securing financing for real estate investments.

7. Historic Preservation and Cultural Heritage

Historic Districts: Respect historic preservation regulations and design guidelines in designated historic districts to preserve architectural heritage, cultural l as landmarks, and historic properties.

Heritage Conservation: Obtain necessary approvals and permits for alterations, renovations, or adaptive reuse projects involving historic properties to ensure compliance with preservation standards as and regulations.

8. Land Use Planning and Development

Comprehensive Plans: Align development with local comprehensive plans, urban growth boundaries, and long-term land. Use goals established by municipal planning departments.

Development Impact Fees: Consider development impact fees, infrastructure requirements, and community benefit contributions associated with new development projects to address the impact on public services and utilities.

9. Homeowners' Association(HOA) Regulations

HOA Covenants: Abide by homeowners' association covenants, conditions, and restrictions (CC&Rs) that govern property use, architectural standards, landscaping, and maintenance requirements in planned communities or condominium complexes.

HOA Fees: Budget for HOA fees, evaluations, and dues imposed by homeowners' association to cover common expenses, amenities, and maintenance.

10. Legal Liability and Insurance Liability Protection: Safeguard assets and reduce legal liabilities through proper entity

structuring, liability insurance coverage, and risk management strategies tailored real estate investments.

Insurance Prerequisites: Get adequate insurance coverage, including property insurance, liability insurance, umbrella policies, and specialized coverage for specific risks (e.g., flood insurance, earthquake insurance). Real estate investors must navigate a complex regulatory landscape encompassing zoning and land use regulations, building codes, environmental laws, landlord -tenant statutes, tax considerations, financing regulations, historic preservation requirements, land use planning, homeowners association rules, legal liability, and insurance requirements. By understanding and complying with regulatory considerations, investors can lessen risks, ensure legal compliance, and optimize the success of their real estate investments.

Diversifying Real Estate Investment Portfolio

Diversifying a real estate investment portfolio involves spreading investment capital across different types of properties, locations, asset classes, and investment strategies to reduce risk, enhance returns, and achieve a balanced portfolio. Here are broad points on how to successfully diversify a real estate investment portfolio effectively:

1. Property Types:

Residential Properties: invest in single-family homes, multi-family apartment buildings, condominiums, townhouses, or vacation rentals to expand exposure to various segments of the housing market. Commercial Properties: Include office buildings, retail centers, industrial warehouses, accommodation properties, and mixed-use developments in your portfolio, to capture income from commercial leases and capitalize on different tenant bases.

Specialized Properties: Consider specialized properties, for example, healthcare facilities, senior housing, self-storage facilities, student housing, or data centers to capitalize on niche market opportunities and unique demand drivers.

2. Geographic Areas:

Regional Diversity: invest in properties located in different geographic regions, cities, states, or countries to mitigate risks associated with economic downturns, regulatory changes, or environmental factors.

Market Dynamics: Assess local market conditions, population growth trends, employment opportunities, infrastructure investments, and economic indicators to identify good investment markets with strong growth potential and favorable risk -returns.

3. Risk Profiles:

Balanced risk exposure: Keep a decent mix of safe, moderate-risk, and high-risk investments in the portfolio to enhance a desired risk-return profile.

Asset Allocation: Decide the appropriate allocation of capital across different asset classes, sectors, and Investment strategies based on investment objectives, risk tolerance, and time horizon.

4. Investment Vehicles

Direct Ownership: Secure physical properties directly through direct ownership or joint ventures to have control over investment decisions, cash flows, and property management.

Real Estate Investment Trusts(REITs): invest in publicly traded REITs or private REITs to gain exposure to expanded portfolios of income-producing properties across different sectors and geographic regions with liquidity, diversification, and professional management.

Real Estate Funds: Consider investing in real estate funds such as private equity funds, hedge funds, or crowdfunding platforms that offer access to professionally managed portfolios of real estate assets with pooled capital from multiple investors.

5. Property Characteristics:

Asset Class Diversification: diversify across different asset classes within real estate, such as residential, commercial, industrial, hospitality, or mixed-use properties, to balance income generation, capital appreciation potential, and risk exposure.

Property Size and Scale: Invest in properties of varying sizes, scales, and asset values, including large-scale institutional-grades properties, mid-size properties, and small-scale properties, to diversify exposure to different market segments and tenant profiles.

6. Cash Flow vs. Appreciation

Income-producing Properties: provides stable cash flows and consistent rental income to provide ongoing income and downside protection during market downturns.

Appreciation Potential: Designate a portion of the portfolio to properties with solid appreciation potential, growth prospects, and value creation opportunities to achieve capital appreciation and long-term wealth accumulation.

7. Portfolio Rebalancing:

Regular Review: Conduct periodic reviews and assessments of the real estate investment portfolio to evaluate performance, rebalance assess performance, rebalance asset allocation, and adjust investment strategies based on changing market conditions, investment objectives, and risk profiles.

Portfolio Optimization: Upgrade the portfolio by reallocation capital to underperforming assets, trimming overvalued assets, and reinvesting in assets with reinvesting in resources with attractive returns to enhance portfolio diversification and maximize long-term returns. Broadening a real estate investment portfolio involves strategic allocation of capital across different property types, geographic locations, risk profiles, investment vehicles, property characteristics, cash flow vs. appreciation considerations, and portfolio rebalancing. By expanding effectively, investors can reduce risks, improve returns, and build a strong portfolio capable of withstanding market volatility and economic uncertainties.

CHAPTER FIVE

Investing in Real Estate Investment Trusts (REITs)

Real Estate Investment Trusts (REITs) are investment vehicles that allow individuals to invest in real estate assets without directly owning or managing properties. REITs pool capital from multiple investors to invest in income-generating real estate properties, including commercial properties, residential complexes, industrial warehouses, retail centers, hospitality properties, and healthcare facilities. Here's an extensive overview of REITs, including their structure, types, benefits, risks, and considerations:

1. Structure and Operation: Legal Structure: REITs are structured as corporations, trusts, or associations that own and operate income-producing real estate properties or finance real estate investments.

2. Tax Status: To qualify as a REIT, a company must meet certain IRS requirements, including distributing at least 90% of its taxable income to shareholders in the form of dividends and investing at least 75% of its assets in real estate.

Ownership: Investors can purchase shares of publicly traded REITs listed on stock exchanges or invest in non-traded REITs through private offerings or direct placements.

Types of REITs:

Equity REITs: Own and operate income-generating properties, collecting rental income and capital appreciation from property investments.

Mortgage REITs (mREITs): Invest in mortgage-backed securities or provide financing for real estate transactions, earning income from interest payments on mortgage loans.

Hybrid REITs: Combine elements of both equity and mortgage REITs, investing in a mix of real estate properties and mortgage-related assets.

Benefits ,,

Diversification: REITs offer exposure to a diversified portfolio of real estate assets across different sectors, geographic locations, and property types, reducing individual property risk.

Liquidity: Publicly traded REITs provide liquidity as shares can be bought and sold on stock exchanges, offering investors flexibility and ease of access to real estate investments.

Income Generation: REITs typically distribute a significant portion of their taxable income to shareholders in the form of dividends, providing a steady stream of income to investors.

Potential for Capital Appreciation: Investors may benefit from capital appreciation as property values increase over time, resulting in higher share prices for equity REITs.

Professional Management: REITs are managed by experienced real estate professionals who handle property acquisition, leasing, management, and disposition, relieving investors of day-to-day management responsibilities.

4. Risks and Considerations:

Market Risk: REITs are subject to market fluctuations, interest rate movements, and economic downturns that can impact property values, rental income, and share prices.

-Liquidity Risk: While publicly traded REITs offer liquidity, non-traded REITs may have limited liquidity and redemption options, making it difficult for investors to sell shares.

Interest Rate Risk: Rising interest rates can increase borrowing costs for REITs, reducing profitability and potentially lowering dividend yields.

Property Risk: REITs are exposed to property-specific risks such as vacancies, tenant defaults, lease expirations, and property damage or deterioration.

Regulatory Risk: Changes in tax laws, regulations, or REIT requirements could affect the tax treatment of REIT dividends or the operational structure of REITs.

5. Due Diligence and Research:

Financial Performance: Evaluate the financial performance of REITs, including dividend yield, funds from operations (FFO), net asset value (NAV), occupancy rates, rental income, and debt levels.

Portfolio Composition: Assess the composition of the REIT's portfolio, including property types, geographic diversification, tenant mix, lease terms, and property quality.

Management Team: Research the experience, track record, and expertise of the REIT's management team in real estate investment, asset management, and property operations.

Industry Outlook: Consider macroeconomic factors, industry trends, and market dynamics that may impact the performance of specific real estate sectors or property types targeted by the REIT.

REITs offer investors an efficient and accessible way to invest in real estate assets, providing diversification, liquidity, income generation, and potential for capital appreciation. However, investors should carefully consider the risks, perform due diligence, and conduct thorough research before investing in REITs to align with their investment objectives, risk tolerance, and financial goals.

Benefits of investing in REITs for wealth accumulation

Investing in Real Estate Investment Trusts (REITs) can offer numerous benefits for wealth accumulation, providing investors with exposure to real estate assets while offering liquidity, diversification, income generation, and potential for capital appreciation. Here's an extensive overview of the benefits of investing in REITs for wealth accumulation:

Diversification.
Asset Diversification: REITs allow investors to diversify their investment portfolios by adding exposure to real estate assets without the need to directly own or manage properties.

Sector Diversification: REITs invest in various sectors of the real estate market, including residential, commercial, retail, industrial, hospitality, and healthcare properties, providing broad diversification across different property types.

Geographic Diversification: REITs may own properties located in different geographic regions, cities, or countries, enabling investors to diversify exposure to regional economic conditions and market dynamics.
2. Income Generation

Steady Dividend Income: REITs are required by law to distribute at least 90% of their taxable income to shareholders in the form of dividends, providing investors with a steady stream of income.

High Dividend Yields: REITs often offer higher dividend yields compared to other asset classes such as stocks or bonds, making them attractive for income-oriented investors seeking reliable cash flow.

3. Potential for Capital Appreciation.

Property Value Appreciation: REITs may benefit from capital appreciation as property values increase over time due to factors such as rising demand, population growth, inflation, or improvements in property fundamentals.

Share Price Appreciation: Investors may realize capital gains through share price appreciation as the market value of REIT shares increases in response to strong financial performance, favorable market conditions, or investor demand.

4. Liquidity:

Publicly Traded REITs: Most REITs are publicly traded on stock exchanges, providing investors with liquidity as shares can be bought and sold easily on the secondary market.

Non-Traded REITs: While non-traded REITs may have limited liquidity compared to publicly traded REITs, they still offer redemption options and liquidity events, providing investors with some degree of flexibility.

5. Professional Management

Experienced Management Teams: REITs are managed by experienced real estate professionals who handle property acquisition, leasing, management, and) disposition, leveraging their expertise to optimize property performance and enhance shareholder value.

Active Asset Management: REIT managers actively manage their portfolios, seeking to maximize rental income, minimize vacancies, optimize property operations, and identify value-enhancing opportunities through strategic acquisitions, development projects, or asset repositioning.

6. Tax Advantages

Pass-Through Taxation: REITs are pass-through entities that pass the majority of their taxable income to shareholders, reducing corporate-level taxation and potentially resulting in higher after-tax returns for investors.

Dividend Tax Treatment: Dividends received from REITs may qualify for favorable tax treatment, including lower tax rates for qualified dividends or the ability to defer taxes through retirement accounts such as IRAs or 401(k)s.

7. Accessibility:

Accessible to All Investors: REITs provide access to real estate investments for individual investors, regardless of their net worth, offering an opportunity to participate in the real estate market with relatively low minimum investment requirements.

Ease of Ownership: Investing in REITs is as simple as buying shares of publicly traded stocks or mutual funds, offering convenience and accessibility for investors seeking exposure to real estate assets.

8. Inflation Hedge:

Inflation Protection: Real estate assets, including those held by REITs, have historically demonstrated resilience against inflationary pressures, as property values

Qualities of good investors

Real estate investors exhibit a diverse range of traits and characteristics that contribute to their success in navigating the complexities of the real estate market.

1. Patience: Successful real estate investors understand that real estate is a long-term investment. They exhibit patience when waiting for the right opportunities to arise, whether it's finding the perfect property, negotiating favorable terms, or waiting for market conditions to align with their investment goals.

2. Financial Literacy: A deep understanding of financial concepts such as cash flow analysis, return on investment (ROI), leverage, and risk management is essential for real estate investors. They can evaluate the financial viability of potential investments, assess risk factors, and make informed decisions to maximize returns.

3. Market Knowledge: Real estate investors stay informed about local market trends, economic indicators, zoning regulations, and demographic shifts. This market knowledge helps them identify emerging opportunities, anticipate changes in property values, and adapt their investment strategies accordingly.

4. Risk Management:

Successful real estate investors are adept at managing risk and mitigating potential pitfalls. They conduct thorough due diligence on properties, assess risk factors such as vacancy rates, tenant quality, and market volatility, and implement strategies to minimize exposure to downside risks.

5. Networking Skills:

Building a strong network of industry professionals, including real estate agents, brokers, contractors, lenders, and property managers, is crucial for real estate investors. Networking provides access to valuable resources, information, and opportunities, enhancing their ability to find and capitalize on lucrative deals.

6. Negotiation Skills:
Negotiation is a fundamental skill for real estate investors, whether it's bargaining with sellers, contractors, or tenants. Successful investors can effectively negotiate terms, prices, and concessions to secure favorable deals and maximize profitability

7. Creativity: Real estate investing often requires creative problem-solving and innovative thinking. Successful investors can adapt to changing market conditions, find unconventional solutions to challenges, and identify opportunities where others may not see them.

8. Persistence: Real estate investing can be challenging and fraught with obstacles, but successful investors remain persistent in pursuing their goals. They are resilient in the face

of setbacks, learn from failures, and persevere until they achieve success.

9. Vision: Successful real estate investors have a clear vision of their investment goals and strategies. Whether it's building a diversified portfolio, achieving financial independence, or revitalizing distressed properties, they have a long-term vision that guides their decision-making and actions.

10. Discipline: Discipline is essential for real estate investors to stay focused on their investment objectives, adhere to budgetary constraints, and follow through on their investment plans. They avoid impulsive decisions, stick to their investment criteria, and maintain a disciplined approach to risk management and portfolio management.

Successful real estate investors possess a combination of patience, financial literacy, market knowledge, risk management skills, networking abilities, negotiation skills, creativity, persistence, vision, and discipline. Cultivating these traits can enhance an investor's ability to identify lucrative opportunities, navigate market fluctuations, and achieve long-term success in real estate investing.

How Does Investing in Real Estate Generate Income?

You can earn money in a variety of ways by investing in real estate, a tried-and-true strategy. The two fundamental techniques are Value appreciation and Rental Income:

- Value Appreciation: Over time, property values have increased. We call this expansion in value appreciation. Any professional would agree that location should be your primary consideration when investing. A neighborhood's perceived desirableness raises property values. Have you heard the expression, "Purchase the most terrible-looking house in the best neighborhood?" There is some truth to this. It's smarter to buy a house you can fix up in a nice neighborhood than an okay house in a terrible area. You can likewise look into investing in an up-and-coming area.

- Rental income: Some real estate investors will only rely on the value of the property rising. For instance, perhaps they live in the property or invest in a vacation home. Notwithstanding, many realtors like to grow their wealth by generating rental income. By leasing the property you own, besides the fact that that property is increasing in value over time, you're earning a monthly income. Your level of involvement ultimately depends on you, however, a few landowners who work with a property manager can label this income as passive.

In an ideal situation, your renters would pay for your mortgage and a portion of your profits. (It'll turn a pure profit once the mortgage is paid off). You must also ensure that maintenance and repairs are included in your budget. If you don't already know how to invest in real estate, breaking into the industry can be intimidating. An investor's confidence and comfort in real estate can take years to develop. That's why beginner-friendly investing strategies are a great place to start. They are suitable for investors with little to no experience, but when properly managed, they can still be extremely profitable. Before taking on more complex investments, it is a great idea to begin in an area of investing that is suitable for beginners. Investors can learn how to raise capital without committing to a deal they may not be able to handle by starting with a simple strategy. This will also help them get to know their local market and build a network. Investors can then move on to other strategies using their experience and profits. For beginners, the following real estate investment strategies can serve as a foundation:

1. Wholesaling: This methodology permits investors to act as a middleman among vendors and purchasers. Wholesalers will identify and secure a property under market value, and afterward assign that contract to an end buyer.

2. Prehabbing: Prehabbing is the most common way of positioning a property for resale by adding minor corrective updates. After that, the property is then often sold to an investor who will carry out a full renovation.

3. REIT Investing: A real estate investment trust(REIT) is an organization that owns and oversees income-producing properties. Investors can then buy shares in REIT and benefit from the productivity of real estate without owning physical properties.

4. Online Real Estate Platforms: Online platforms help to connect investors with real estate developers. In exchange for

monthly or quarterly repayments, including interest, the investors contribute to the financing of real estate projects.

In a nutshell, the following is a comprehensive summary of what a novice in real estate investment should know:

.Understanding Real Estate Investment: Real estate involves buying, owning, managing, renting, or selling real estate for profit.

. Types of Real Estate: Residential (single-family homes, condos, apartments), Commercial (offices, buildings, retail spaces), Industrial (warehouses, factories), and Land (undeveloped property).

. Investing Strategies

- Buy and Hold: Buying a property to rent it out for long-term income and the possibility of appreciation

- Fix and Flip: Purchasing distressed properties, renovating them, and selling them for profit.

- Real Estate Investment Trusts (REITs): Real estate-related investments in publicly traded businesses.

- Real Estate Crowdfunding: Pooling funds with other investors to invest in real estate projects.

Market Analysis: To make informed investment decisions, and research local market trends, property values, rental rates, and economic indicators.

. Financing Options: Options incorporate mortgages, hard money loans, private lenders, partnerships, or using your funds.

. Risk Management: Consider factors like market unpredictability, tenant turnover, property maintenance, and monetary slumps.

. Property Management: Choose whether to self-manage or hire a property management company to deal with everyday operations, tenant relations, and maintenance. Exit Strategies: Plan for how to liquidate or divest from investments if necessary, like selling, refinancing, or passing down properties.

. Continuous Learning: Read books, take courses, attend seminars, and network with other investors to stay updated on industry trends, regulations, and market conditions. Real estate thorough research, financial planning, and risk management. It can be lucrative but also comes with risk, so it's essential to approach it with careful consideration and diligence.

Conclusion

For novices willing to navigate its complexities, real estate investment presents a wealth-building opportunity. By grasping the different investment strategies, conducting thorough market analysis, and managing risks effectively. Investors can build an expanded portfolio that generates recurring, automated income and long term appreciation. It's significant for amateurs to grasp the legal, financial, and tax considerations handle on the lawful, monetary, related with real estate investment, as well as to remain informed about industry patterns and guidelines. In addition, forming a network of professionals and fellow investors can offer helpful advice and encouragement along the way. While real estate investment offers the potential for significant returns, it's not without its difficulties. Investors must be able to adapt to changes in the market, effectively manage properties, and continuously educate themselves in order to make well-informed decisions. At last, outcome in real estate investment requires persistence, determination, and an eagerness to gain from both successes and failures. Beginners in real estate investment can embark on a rewarding journey toward financial independence with careful planning, diligence, and a long-term mindset.

www.ingramcontent.com/pod-product-compliance
Lightning Source LLC
Chambersburg PA
CBHW070409230526
45471CB00006B/2722